Autistic Shoes

Evolution of Behaviour

Andrew Brown

British Library Cataloguing In Publication Data
A Record of this Publication is available
from the British Library

ISBN 978-1-84685-621-1

First Published 2007 by
Exposure Publishing,
an imprint of
Diggory Press Ltd
Three Rivers, Minions, Liskeard, Cornwall, PL14 5LE, UK
and of Diggory Press, Inc.,
Goodyear, Arizona, USA
WWW.DIGGORYPRESS.COM

Contents

Part One

The Evolution common human behaviour and the formation of Original and Tribal minds

Part Two

What our Evolution means to us Today

Foreword

I first came across autistic spectrum disorder two and a half years ago through a series of unfortunate events. I am not going to describe what happened; it just suffices to say that the disorder happened upon my doorstep and created a war of understanding. It has to be said the battles I have waged were like frontal assaults straight into a warm plate of soft blanc-mange. In the interests of my own sanity I needed to find an explanation for behaviour that might seem unusual but not abnormal and certainly not in my view constituting any mental disorder. When I started to look at a particular description at the high functioning end of the autistic spectrum I could see a pattern. The pattern I saw was not one of disorder but of characteristics missing that would come from a tribe.

This set me thinking perhaps our perceptions are wrong. Maybe the autistic personality isn't what we think it is. I looked at the specifics of something called Asperger's Syndrome, which is classed as a disorder on the autistic spectrum. I thought current understanding doesn't seem right and when you see where it comes from you will see why it isn't. All the problems listed are simply observations of missing tribal characteristics. These people don't have a disorder at all they simply didn't come from a tribe. The characteristics they do have would come from evolution in a single-family. This in turn gave me a vision of our world. It is not as we see it. We as a species are made up from two personalities.

I do recognise that many people perhaps rely on a diagnosis of mental disorder for protection of their children in school. I feel that this says rather more about the lack of ability of the school rather than any problem with the child. What I want to show you is the reason why we behave in different ways and for the answer I have turned to evolutionary psychology. From my initial observations I have worked backwards and forwards through time to get things to fit together. I wanted to be able to place our characteristics in an order that made sense. As well as the characteristics that make us different I wanted to establish the ones that we all have in common. I consider this to be important because from it we can establish what to expect. To get to this I have gone all the way back to the start of evolution. This has in the end given me a picture that makes sense. It may not be a perfect drawing but I think you will recognise it when you see it.

I am not all alone in my notion. In 1998 a man named Nicholas Humphrey touched on the same thing in a paper called *"Cave art, autism, and evolution of the human mind"*. He observed astonishing parallels between prehistoric cave art and drawings by an autistic child. In his paper he makes the following proposal: *"The makers of these works of art may actually have had distinctly pre-modern minds, have been little given to symbolic thought, have had no great interest in communication and have been essentially self-taught and untrained. Cave art, so far from being the sign of a new order of mentality, may perhaps be thought the swan-song of old."*

His choice of expression in the term *"pre-modern"* is not accurate. *"Pre-tribal"* would be the correct term. I also find the very term *"autistic"* itself not the best description available for this mind. A much better and more accurate term would be the *"original mind"*. It has in fact been integral to human development and has only recently been reduced in status to mentally disordered. It in reality created the modern world. I find that the term *"disability"* is not the best description available for protecting this mind. A better term would be *"different ability"*. It can be more or less able and in fact is just as likely to suffer problems the cleverer it is because then it creates fear.

"Autistic shoes" is written mainly in the style of a story however it is not just a story. My intention is to try and be of interest to everybody with the main point of reference being you and me. I feel that one thing I cannot be

accused of is lacking imagination but then maybe it is not just my imagination. We have set expectations of things. Scientists give us progress. Psychologists tell us if we are normal. Religious leaders tell us God's will. Now what if that essence of God within ourselves were far more powerful than the people of status in which we trust. Well then we might find something different we might in fact find truth.

Chapter One

Introduction

This is a quote by Charles Darwin from the *"Origin of Species"*. *" In the distant future I see open fields for far more important researches. Psychology will be based on a new foundation, that of the necessary acquirement of each mental power and capacity by gradation. Light will be thrown on the origin of man and his history"*. (Darwin, 1859, p.458 Origin of Species).

This is a quote about Darwin's notion of natural selection published some forty years after the *"Origin of Species"* *"How extremely stupid not to have thought of that!"*(T.Huxley, 1900 p.170 Life and Letters of Thomas Henry Huxley, Vol 1. London: Macmillan). This quote I believe aptly applies to this work however I hope it will take a little less time for someone to say it again.

I intend to set out the path of human evolution from pretty much the start of conscious thought. This is an ambitious project you may say. It has been over one hundred and fifty years since Darwin's "Origin of Species" and I haven't seen as yet a concise story of human evolution that makes real sense. Why should one come now you ask?

The reason is circumstance. A key piece of research was first published in 1944 but didn't really come to light until the 1980's. This research like Darwin's was one of observation but of human behaviour. The work was in my view erroneous in its conclusions in so far as it identified something being wrong. What it did identify however was a human mind alive now that had not evolved natural social characteristics that most people consider to be normal. I say most people however as I sit here in Wales these characteristics seem to be rather more normal than people make out.

The fundamental idea that I use to find the story of human evolution is this. We have been formed by evolution and it is those evolutionary experiences that give us the body and mind we have today. This being the case we can use our body and minds to unravel evolution and find where we came from. In other words as Darwin put it we can *"throw light on the origin of man and his history"*.

Although our body provides glimpses of our past history it is our mind that contains the clearest record of how we were made. Each one of us comes complete with instructions of how we worked through evolution a bit like a users manual. Until now we haven't been able to read the manual because it has been in a language we haven't fully recognised. We are going to translate it. This translation will probably not be perfect but hopefully a bit better than the one that came with the instruction manual for my Chinese motorcycle. This is a short quote *" Thank you for your purchase of motorcycle. We will express our sincere thanks to you for your wisc choose. We believe our motorcycle will serve you comfortably with its elegant. Up-to-date structure and excellent performance. Through various tests and driving it has proved to be of good performance. They are really ideal transportation means of modern people because of luxurious appearance, bcomfortable in riding and easy and safe in operation"* I am not sure I made quite such a wisc choose but there you are.

Does understanding our evolutionary story have any relevance other than simply being of interest? It does. If we want to understand psychology or how people think and behave we need to understand our evolutionary story. For instance I recently visited an old lead mine near Aberystwyth. As we went down the mine one little girl was screaming with terror in the dark of the narrow passageways. To a friend who was with me this was a bit annoying. The little girl's parents weren't altogether too pleased. To me it was completely understandable. I knew why she was screaming and what she was terrified of.

More fundamentally our evolutionary story can reveal to us what is normal to expect in human behaviour. This behaviour is not the same for everybody. At the moment I perceive the profession of psychology as a little embryonic in its understanding of the human mind. It classes some types of behaviour as dysfunction or disorder as though something is wrong. We are in a position to dispel those old views. I am not a psychologist. I have not been rampaging around diagnosing this that and the other and hence have no previous preconceptions to take account of. I can present to you what I believe is the truth. In my view the most therapeutic aspect of a visit to the shrink occurs when they are less sane than you. At least you can think well I am not that bonkers. There is a more serious side however to problems with some of our previous psychology research into human behaviour. We have inherited work based on the false foundations of eugenics and we will later in the book take a more detailed look at this.

Normally you might expect the story of human evolution to come from a professor after years of research. This is not the person that such a story will come from. The reason is the nature of academic study. People specialise in narrow fields of expertise. I have seen attempts at trying to get academics from different fields to cooperate together however I think we know what tends to come out of committees. We are going to look right across the board to find the evidence that gives us our evolutionary story. This evidence will include psychology, physiology, paleoanthropology, mythology, dreams, human physical activity, sexual behaviour, religion, environmental change and most likely some others on our way.

I am going to take you right back to the time that the first creatures evolved in the sea and emerged on to land. This will be a journey through our human fears. I will show you an early human evolution driven by fear. I will explain how each fear developed our instincts. This journey back through time will take us from water to dry land. It will take us from day into night and then back into day again. It takes us from living on the ground to under the ground to living above the ground and back to the ground again. Remnants of all these lifestyles are left in our body and behaviour.

We will progress through the time we evolved as hominoids following our descent from the trees. We will look at how hominoid physical and mental characteristics of our ancestors developed. We will link evolution to environmental change with the onset of ice age and how through the environment the single human family evolved. We will follow the changing environment to the establishment of the tribe. There is however a twist in the tale. This twist will lead us to the formation of the modern world, as we know it today. The twist is that the human world is not formed out of a single type of human mind. The modern world is formed out of two distinctly separate types of basic human mind. One is a descendant of the other.

I talk of "we" taking an evolutionary journey. This is you and me. I am merely a guide on our travels. Our mode of transport will be mathematical. We are going to use the process of logic to find our way. I will set out logical reasons for things and you will judge whether you think that is right or not. You will be the judge and the jury. Am I telling the truth?

Chapter Two

The five concepts we will use to understand our evolution

There are five basic concepts I have established that help us understand human evolution. From these concepts we can establish a way of thinking that explains how our evolutionary experiences are reflected in ourselves today. These concepts are:

1) The concept of the compression of evolutionary time into a single point in our minds
2) The concept of human ancestry in a different physical form and size to ourselves.
3) The concept of evolutionary experience being laid in layers in our mind.
4) The concept group structures we recognise today coming from different phases in evolution.
5) The concept of the most competitive creatures holding the original central territory

The concept of evolutionary time compression

The concept that has enabled me to take us back to the early days of human evolution is the concept of the compression of evolutionary time. It needs to be born in mind that we have been formed over some 3 or 4 billion years although conscious thought is a bit more recent than that. This time scale however is not contained by the human mind in a linear fashion as we conventionally think of time rather it is compressed into a single point. Human characteristics that we inherited say 150,000 years ago function alongside characteristics that we inherited 200 million years ago. As I go through the story I talk of evolution from any time period as though it were yesterday because that is how we need to think of evolution. 200

13

million years ago is no more distant to our minds than is yesterday. It would be true to say that the more complex human characteristics came later, as we became more complex organisms. However the characteristics still remain from early evolution functioning along side those later characteristics in the single time frame of now in the living mind.

We will use the concept of the compression of evolutionary time to explore the human fears we have. This will allow us to travel back to any point in time and let us to think of it as yesterday. We can make real sense of our fears.

The concept of the different human form

If you think of the whole of evolution from the single cell to what we are today there has been a range in size and form from microscopic to what we are now. It is a case of taking ourselves back to the size and form we were at certain points in time to make sense of our history. We have not always been like we are now.

For instance people say to me that man didn't exist at the time of the dinosaurs and that is true in terms of the way we think of ourselves in our present physical form. We were not walking around upright or even had the form of a primate like creature. However we did exist because we have existed since the start of life its self. What I am asking you to consider is this. Disregard our current physical form and try and imagine us in a form that has changed through evolution. Even in recent times we have physically changed. We have grown taller on average for instance in the last few hundred years. The process of evolution is one of gradual change from one generation to the next. When comparing one creature to its ancestry over many generations we can have significant change. The human ancestors may be your several millionth great grandfathers and grandmothers however I am proposing that we try and recognise them as the same creatures as

14

we would recognise ourselves. They may have been perhaps in some mouse like creature or frog like form but you have inherited evolutionary experiences that they had.

The concept of the evolutionary layering of the mind

Charles Darwin uses the term *"by capacity of gradation"* in the way he establishes the concept of evolution. This term means a series of gradual successive changes that give rise to an overall change and a creature evolving from one form to another. This process however does not happen at a constant pace. The pace of change is variable dependant on circumstance. The effect of this is to leave layers or general phases of evolution. At a time of evolutionary pressure for survival relatively rapid change occurs. At a time of little evolutionary pressure little change occurs. These layers of change can be seen in the human mind and body today.

I am proposing that the human mind is layered with evolutionary programming like the strata of rock from an ancient riverbed. This concept is not to be taken in the physical sense literally. There are some physical identifiable differences in the brain from evolution. For instance the part that controls fear is near the core and as such was likely to have been formed in early evolution. I wish to take the mind as a whole entity and consider it as layers of programming one laid on top of the other. The earlier layers are written over and may be clouded but crucially they are not lost. In this way we can understand our diverse range in behaviour. For instance it explains the range in human sexual behaviour. Promiscuity was established at one period or phase in evolution. Monogamy was established at another phase in evolution. Both layers of behavioural programming function together in the living human mind.

15

The concept of human group structures from different phases of evolution

It is human group structure that tells us how the later part of our evolution occurred. Taking the concept layering of the mind and different behavioural programming coming from different phases we can establish the specifics of this evolution. These specifics centre on the existence of two forms of human group behaviour. The first of these forms is the existence of the single human family consisting of a man a woman and children. The other form is that of the existence of the tribal group consisting of several families. Each came from different times in evolution.

The crucial research that Darwin was missing comes in here. A certain group of human beings did not develop the layer of evolutionary programming from the tribal phase of evolution. Instead these people kept the natural instructions from a single-family existence. The research established that these people still exist. Through the process of logic we can place the single-family at an earlier phase in human evolution than tribal group existence. Had the tribe come first then everybody would have tribal group social characteristics and they don't.

The research I refer to was first published in 1944 and forms the basis of what is currently termed Asperger's Syndrome, which is classified as an autistic spectrum disorder. We will later run through the characteristics of this personality using it to explain evolution and evolution to explain it.

The concept of the most competitive creatures holding the original central territory

Throughout the story of human evolution I use this concept to establish the ancestors home. This home originates in East Africa the birthplace of humanity and our story centres on the location of the Great Rift Valley. We can deduce for instance that we were the most competitive hominoid because we were the last out of Africa and we are the only one surviving today. Through our evolution however we have not always been the most competitive of creatures and this has driven us to various homes. We have not always held the original central territory but have been pushed out through competition to the periphery at certain times in our past.

The concept will further be used to explain the pattern of human migration out of Africa. We will have waves of migrations based on relative competitiveness. The most competitive hold the original central territory the longest. Further more this concept will help us explain the very pattern of civilisation its self. We will see the reason for the unusual locations that civilisation occurred in. Finally some light may be cast on the general geographical pattern of the modern human world today.

Chapter Three

Human evolution driven by inferiority

Rather than man's ancestors being the most competitive of creatures this story is based on the ancestors being inferior creatures. It is by being inferior that evolution was forced along the route it took and change occurred as a matter of necessity in the battle for survival. This inferiority would eventually lead to superiority through the process of natural selection. The weaker creatures were weeded out to give us the fine specimen of humanity we have today.

John Roach reported in the National Geographic News on 4th October 2001 on research carried out by a psychologist called Arne Ohman and his colleagues at the Karolinska Institute and Hospital in Stockholm, Sweden. This research suggests that fear of snakes and spiders, has been shaped by evolution, stretching back to a time when early mammals had to survive and breed in an environment dominated by reptiles, some of which were deadly. Joseph LeDoux, a professor of neural science and psychology at New York University said that Arne Ohman's work was generally accepted in the scientific community. "Certainly there are certain stimuli that are pre-wired in the brain because they have been perennially dangerous to our ancestors".

Now I am going to take this idea and expand it. I believe that these creatures were not merely dangerous but were predators on our several millionth great grand parents. Those creatures were superior and we were lunch. Their superiority meant our inferiority and consequently deep-rooted fears evolved out of this inferiority in the battle for survival. There are creatures today that are dangerous that we are not afraid of. The most dangerous is the mosquito, however are we afraid when we see a mosquito land and bite us on our arm? It is by being eaten that we become so afraid not merely by the relative danger of a creature.

The idea that fears are inherited isn't recent. The father of evolutionary theory Charles Darwin himself made this proposition in the following words *"May we not suspect that the vague but very real fears of children, which are quite independent of experience, are inherited effects of real dangers and abject superstitions during ancient savage times"*. These fears are etched in the human mind and are all there to be unravelled. In doing so prehistoric evolution can be unravelled. Fear has all arisen out of sustained and substantial traumatic events of such magnitude that they became etched as a basic survival blueprint on the human ancestors. It was the ancestors that developed these fears that survived and we in turn have inherited them. It is by considering the pre-primate human form that the earliest fears make sense. Size is the critical issue to consider and this is from when we were tiny creatures.

Darwin's proposition of *"vague but very real fears of children"* is the proposition that we are going to follow. Children pass through the whole evolutionary process as they grow. The human embryo encapsulates our earliest evolution. We start off as a single cell, which is just how we started in evolution along with all other life forms. The embryo resembles an aquatic creature in early pregnancy. Babies start out with no concept of fear just as we had no concept of fear right at the beginning of time. As the baby grows into the child so the fears become apparent. Monsters, the dark and bogie men prey on the young child's mind. All these things were killers at one time or another in our evolution and the young child re-lives those times in his bed at night. I hope we will have a little more sympathy when we think just how terrifying our early history was.

We shall therefore layout the order in which these fears evolved. This is the "Order of Fear"

The order of fear

Fear of being eaten

Fear of water

Fear of spiders

Fear of monsters.

Fear of the dark, tight spaces and snakes.

Fear of heights

Fear of the bogie man

I hope this list wets your appetite for the journey ahead. If by chance you are thinking what an earth is he going on about then read on and see. We are going back in time to a life dominated by fear.

Part One

The Evolution of common human behaviour and the formation of Original and Tribal minds

Chapter Four

The beginning of human evolution and life driven by fear

In the beginning single cells were created and some of these cells cooperated together and so was created the patch of slime. Now I don't want you to think that this is the end of evolution even though this perhaps resembles your line manager at work or somebody else you know. Higher life forms would evolve and in time began to gain the process of conscious thought. Those that thought stood a better chance of survival. With the process of thought came the basic mental programming of creatures. This programming was for the purposes of survival and involved the need to eat and reproduce.

It is from this point in evolution that we have inherited our most basic sexual programming. This programming is bisexual although it wasn't at the time because there was only one sex. There were no males or females we were basically similar in make up to perhaps a worm. This sexual programming is still evident today in homosexuality. On the face it of homosexuality serves no evolutionary purpose. Couples of the same sex cannot produce offspring and hence this behaviour should die out. The reason homosexuality doesn't die out is because we are all basically bisexual. It is from this point in evolution that bisexuality served evolutionary purpose and we have all inherited this most basic sexual attraction to each other. I observe my chickens trying to mate with each other when there is no cockerel around. My dog does it with other dogs. Young bulls do it with each other and so do the ram lambs. Bisexuality will be common to all creatures and is the basis for sexual behaviour. And by the way if you are thinking have I done it I haven't. My later evolutionary programming has proved dominant.

Eventually creatures would evolve that ate other creatures. The creatures that were eaten evolved and the next level of mental programming came to be. This was the evolution of fear.

Fear is the first characteristic that can be used to find the specifics of human evolution. The most basic fear is that of being eaten. This evolved in the sea and is common to many creatures. The first specific fear that we can use to track human evolution is that fear that drove us out of the sea on to dry land. I find man's distant ancestor was an amphibian. This amphibian came onto land because of competition in the water. It found itself being eaten by more successful water born predators. The predation on the human ancestor caused a fear and this was the fear of water. A more accurate description really would be a fear of the creatures actually in the water. When you think about it there are a multitude of untold nasty creatures in the sea. There are jellyfish, octopus, sea anemones and squids to name a few and they aren't very nice. Our memories of these creatures have been very clouded indeed by time. This is to the extent that we have various sea creatures particularly with tentacles that make us react with revulsion; however a specific individual predator cannot be identified. The effect of this is reflected in a general inherited fear of water.

I believe that the ancestors of all land born creatures developed a fear of water and it was this that propelled them onto land. When I look forward in time I find it difficult to identify why a land animal would need to go into water sufficiently often to develop fear. I return to my basic cause of fear and that is an exposure to sustained and substantial traumatic events of a magnitude sufficient for that fear to become etched on the mind. The fear of water is expressed in children and there is a reluctance to enter water until they have learned it is safe. Many land animals show a reluctance to enter water. I therefore think this fear is derived from almost the beginning of time when man's ancestor lived in the water.

Through our time in the sea and the evolution of fear we also evolved sexually. As we became more complex organisms driven by competition we split into male and female. This would lead to the next layer of sexual programming and that is sexual attraction to the opposite sex. We would in general find members of the opposite sex more attractive than those of the same sex. Through the splitting of the sexes much more complex organisms would evolve and we were one of these organisms.

Around three or four hundred million years ago the first creatures started to take to land and along with them at some point our several hundred millionth great grand parents. On land we evolved and developed our first distinguishable fear of a particular creature. This creature was the spider. Why the spider you may ask? The reason is two fold.

Spiders are thought to be amongst the earliest animals to live on land. Spiders are predators. A three hundred million year old fossil has been found of a spider-like ancient arachnid. This creature was half a meter long and had massive jaws. It had a shield like cover over its abdomen for protection. I would guess that it inherited its protection from its sea born ancestors, which just goes to show that even worse creatures lived in the sea. Spiders being some of the first creatures on land would gain evolutionary advantage by being first. They would be better adapted to land living than perhaps our ancestors when they emerged from the sea. Looking at spider evolution we can tell they were not especially fast or particularly good at catching things. If they had been they would not have evolved the use of webs. Any way the spider forced our evolution along the route of evasion. The identifiable fear of spiders we have means that the spider was a significant predator to us in our early evolutionary form. The fear we developed of this predator served the purpose of causing us to keep well out of the spider's way. Those that developed the fear stood a better chance of survival.

The fear of spiders still makes us react in the same way today because that fear is etched in the early part of our mind. This part of our mind has no concept of the size we are now. To it we are the same size as we were when this fear was formed. We still steer well clear of spiders and remove them from our houses. As for those people that flush them down the plughole I think they should realise that there is nothing to be afraid of anymore and they can climb back up again anyway.

The second reason I believe that the spider is the earliest recognisable predator we faced is the degree to which our memories of this creature are clouded. For these memories I am looking to mythology. Mythology might be disregarded scientifically however I believe that it provides insight into ancient human memories. The myths themselves may be implausible stories however the subjects they are about are based on reality. When I look at the myths about spiders they appear as both a creature associated with fear but also as a protector.

In myth spiders wove webs to hide David from King Saul, a Japanese warrior called Yoritomo from his enemies and even Mohammed from his enemies. It seems most people had a friendly spider. However this does not make sense. How can a feared creature be a friend? I believe this is because the memories of what the spider actually did to us are so old they are very clouded indeed. The fear is clear however the reason for it is only dimly remembered. This degree of clouding is reflected in the modern day equivalent of myths and these are comic book superheroes. One of these heroes is Spider Man. Again we have a creature of fear acting as protector. The final creature of fear we faced in our early evolution, which we will come to in time, is much better remembered for the losses it inflicted on our ancestors. This creature would not be created into a super hero character because we haven't forgotten what it did to us.

Further creatures would evolve more successfully than the ancestors of man and these creatures would be reptiles. They would become relatively much larger than the human ancestor and would become predators. This would lead to the evolution of a new fear and to a new living environment.

Chapter Five

Our fears and instincts from the time of the dinosaurs

This was a time when reptiles were the top predators. The ancestors of mammals were still small insignificant creatures of which our ancestor was one. The reptiles held the best territory and our ancestors were pressed out to inferior territory. This territory was the rocky outcrops and a place that the superior predators didn't come. The reason behind this location is recorded in a fear we have inherited. The fear the ancestor developed that drove him to his rocky home was the fear of monsters.

Monsters as we think of them now haven't existed since the time of the dinosaurs in terms of size. When we consider relative size and by that I mean the human ancestor being the size of a mouse or perhaps smaller many reptiles would have seemed like monsters and they were to the ancestor. Looking at more recent human evolution I don't think there is an opportunity to develop this fear later than this. If we consider the time of the so far known evolution of the hominoid there is insufficient size difference between the top predators and man's ancestor to really consider these creatures as monsters. They may have been larger than their descendents, which are the big cats and canines of today but they were still not monster size. Children fear monsters and are basically remembering a fear that man's ancestor developed at the time of the dinosaurs. They have inherited this fear from him and perhaps even the images of the monsters he saw.

Man's ancestor lived in the rocky outcrop environment and in this place he developed an ability that would later in evolution lead us to a home where we would develop our primate form. The ability the ancestor developed at this time in evolution was the ability to climb on the rock faces.

The ancestor would travel down from the rock faces to find food and back up again to safety.

Climbing is a bizarre hazardous activity, which on the face of it serves no purpose. Once a climber reaches the top of a cliff or mountain he just comes down again having expended rather a lot of energy in the process. The instinct to climb rocks however is inherited and cannot be denied. We have this instinct although it has been curtailed somewhat by a fear we developed later in evolution which we will come to in due course. Some people however still exercise this ancient instinct in the recreational activity they undertake and that is the activity of rock climbing. It is interesting to note that perhaps the most obvious feature for a primate to climb is a tree. Tree climbing however is not a common recreational activity except amongst children yet rock climbing is. The reason for this is that man evolved climbing abilities on rocks rather than trees. He could already climb when he took to the trees and we indulge the climbing instinct in the place we learnt to climb and that was on rocks.

For an idea of the food the ancestor ate we can look at our teeth for clues. Primates have canine teeth however these teeth are not from living on a diet of fruit. Canine teeth serve no function in this kind of diet. These teeth come from earlier evolution when we were insectivores or small carnivores. The food the ancestor ate probably included insects, snails, and worms and in fact anything that was small and easy to catch.

As evolution progressed so the reptiles evolved into the later dinosaurs. It is from this time I believe we can deduce more detail of a specific monster we feared. This creature evolved to be able to access our rocky outcrop home and we found ourselves no longer safe from the monsters out in the open. This would lead to a new home in the rocks.

Today the most well known dinosaur that we recognise as a monster would be the Tyrannosaurus Rex. We have to however transport ourselves back to the time of the dinosaurs and think of ourselves then. Would the T Rex or some similar older creature have been the monster we feared. I suspect not except for the fact he may have trodden on us occasionally. For an idea of the monster I believe we need to look again to mythology.

The monster that stands out in mythology is the dragon. This is a mythical creature that appears in numerous cultures spread throughout the world. Here in Wales it is the national emblem on the Welsh flag. The dragon is a well-known feature in Chinese culture and most people will have seen pictures of the Chinese dragon. There are dragons from the very birthplace of humanity itself in Ethiopia, East Africa. This dragon myth is known as "The Ethiopian Dream" and the creature has four wings and two feet with claws. The widespread concept of the dragon suggests to me that the dragon is a common memory relevant to all humans and came from a common ancestor.

As we recognise the dragon today it seems impossible for this creature to have ever existed. However I believe it did exist and it is not a simple figment of the imagination. Taking the basic characteristics of the dragon we have a reptile like creature with wings. The question is did any such creature ever exist with these basic characteristics? The answer is yes they did. These creatures came from the time of the dinosaurs and they were Pterosaurs or the flying dinosaurs. It has to be born in mind that in terms of relative size they would have been monsters to our ancestors.

Imagine looking up from the ground as a mouse like being at such a creature. Could this be where we get our vision of a dragon? Imagine being backed into a crevice with a Pterosaur's long beak like jaw with serrated teeth poking in trying to grab you. In the close confines of the hiding place you feel the heat of the breath of this monster it feels like fire. You look out and can see the monsters wings folded as he probes your hiding place trying to find you. Could this be the dragon? We have inherited our ancestor's fears as part of our own fears. We recognise the monsters that our ancestors recognised. These fears and monsters may seem far-fetched now however they weren't at the time. They were real fears and based on real monsters.

Today there are no Pterosaurs to actually see however there is a creature with one of its characteristics and that is the flying dinosaurs wing. This creature may be small however the characteristics of its wings still access the basic human fear of the dragon. The creature is the bat. Now there is no reason for us to fear bats but we do. They are associated with evil and one of the most well known connections is with vampires and Dracula. It is the wing characteristic of the bat that we fear, which comes from this point in evolution the fangs would come latter. This wing is similar to the Pterosaurs wing. There are no feathers just stretched smooth skins. Now if you have ever had a bat flapping around your bedroom you will know just how disconcerting the motion of a bat's wings are. I have tried to catch them to put them outside and find that every time a bat flies close to me I flinch away. This is a natural reaction and stems from evolution. We evolved to fear this wing motion not from bats but from Pterosaurs.

The degree to which our memories of the dragon are clouded is much less so than our memories of the spider. There is a clearer link with an actual monster like creature. Having said this we have still forgotten to a certain degree what this creature did to us. This is reflected in the way we have created a super hero character out of the main characteristics of the dragon and those are its wings. This comic book super hero is Bat Man probably the best-known super hero character of them all. This is by no mere coincidence because the dragon was the last main predator on our ancestors whose deeds have been forgotten sufficiently for this creature to be imbued with protector status.

The fear of monsters and our need to avoid them gives us another human behavioural characteristic that we have inherited and can see today. This characteristic is the desire to hide and is particularly expressed by children. Children crawl under beds, into wardrobes and under tables. They will hide when they are scared. They will hide for fun. They love hiding. The natural desire to hide could come from later in evolution however I think the basic instinct was formed at this point. The characteristics of hiding are all about finding dark inaccessible places.

The instinct to hide leads us to our new home in the rocks and this was in the depths of the crevice. These depths were a place of safety away from the probing beak jaws of the monsters. The ancestors that developed the ability to hide in the depths of the crevice were the ones that survived and passed that ability on to their children.

Humans have inherited the instinct to crawl into the crevices. This instinct can be seen in the way that people make recreation out of potholing. Potholing again is an activity, which is rather strange. People crawl down small cracks in the earth only to eventually come out again usually wetter and more tired than when they went in. Children display the ancient instinct to crawl into the crevice and love crawling through pipes and tubes that are provided in indoor play areas. This instinct to crawl into crevices is an ancient instinct from the time that it served the purpose of evolutionary survival for the ancestor of man. We have inherited this instinct.

The underground instinct also serves a practical purpose in the modern world and that is for the purpose of mining. If you have ever been down a coal mine as I have you will find there is a strange feeling of security. On the face of it a mine would seem a most unnatural place to work. There is however the ancient human instinct from below the ground that makes a mine an anciently natural place to be.

31

This arises from the time we lived in our underground home.

There are other remnants of this underground home left in our behaviour today. We still do not like sleeping out in the open. We use tents, live in buildings and huts. These structures do provide practical purpose in keeping the rain off however they serve a more fundamental evolutionary purpose. That purpose is to recreate our rocky crevice home. This home provided us with safety from the dragons. We have created our huts and houses to cater for this ancient instinct. We still feel the need for the protection of the crevice although the dragons have gone. To this ancient part of our mind however the dragons are still here.

One of the earliest associations we have with death developed at this time. This association is with passage into the skies. The flying reptiles came out of the sky and returned to the sky carrying us with them. This early link between the sky and death would be developed later into the concept of stars being ancestors and even heaven itself being in the skies. The concept of rising up to the heavens through death had its origins in real events that happened in evolution.

By this time in evolution we had evolved into our warm blooded mammalian form. This form allowed us to adapt our behaviour. This meant that we could not only function in the day but we could also function when the heat of the day had gone. This meant we could become creatures of the night.

Chapter Six

We become creatures of the night

The fear of monsters along with his evolution to a mammalian form altered the ancestor's behaviour and he became nocturnal. The reptiles weren't as active at night as they were cold blooded. The Pterosaurs weren't active at all because they relied on clear vision of daylight to fly as well as the heat of the day for their bodies to function. Inferior predators can be seen working at night like the domestic cat. This type of behaviour serves to avoid capture by superior predators. The human mind has retained some of the nocturnal behaviour from this point in evolution. People do not go to sleep as soon as it gets dark. In contrast to this if you observe the behaviour of a chicken you will see that they do go to sleep as soon as it gets dark. This creature is a descendent of the dinosaurs and hasn't evolved to be nocturnal. People today have various nocturnal activities and this behaviour stems from an early nocturnal lifestyle.

One such nocturnal activity that people undertake is sex. The time we generally have sex is quite unusual. Some people do undertake this activity in the day but in general it is at night. We might put this down to our working and so there isn't practical time for it. However I do not think that is the real reason for sexual activity in the night. This nocturnal activity stems from a nocturnal lifestyle. We hadn't evolved any concept of the family or group behaviour at this point in evolution. It was pretty much every mouse for himself and herself. We didn't return to the wife in the rock crevice home after work. We all lived separately. The females reared young without input from the males apart from the sex bit. Nocturnal sex came from nocturnal hunting activity. As well as finding food we would occasionally come across members of the opposite sex in the night. There would be a quick sexual encounter and then back to work.

33

It would be the combination of the ancestor's mammalian physical form, small size and nocturnal life style that would ensure survival through the cataclysm 65 million years ago that wiped out the dinosaurs. The current consensus is that a huge meteor from outer space struck the world with devastating consequences for much of life on earth. In the period after the cataclysm the world was a dark cold and austere place to live. It would be thousands of years before the sun managed to properly shine through the blanket of dust that encapsulated the earth. This environment suited those plants and creatures that could live with a limited intensity of light. Man's ancestor was one of those creatures. He was a creature of the night and was capable of surviving in the new environment.

The crevice was home and the ancestor worked by night. The depths of the crevice had been safe for millennia of time however there was now a predator that had evolved its behaviour to specialise in hunting our ancestors. Even the depths of the crevice were no longer safe. In fact the depths of the crevice were to become a place of fear and death. This place was now a trap with no escape. Once the crevice had been a place of protection but not any longer. An evil creature would enter our homes and kill us in our beds.

The evil creature had evolved through the time of the dinosaurs and had now become the ancestor's greatest foe. It had evolved physically in a way that it was capable of entering the crevices of rocks to hunt us down. It had had a narrow girth but still retained strength through its long body. It had even lost it limbs and could squeeze through the tightest of gaps. The predation on the human ancestor by this creature would leave a number of deeply engrained fears. Those that developed the fears survived.

The first of these fears I want to look at is claustrophobia or the fear of tight spaces. This fear I believe came from the crevice that was home to the human ancestor. To my mind this is the only place to develop such a fear. Looking through the whole of human evolution I have placed it in the time of the caveman but it does not fit. It seems implausible that sufficient traumatic events could occur to cause this fear then. This fear I am certain came from the only other time we lived in a tight space and that was in the crevice at a time earlier in evolution. The fear served the purpose of selecting the human ancestors that evolved the mental desire to have an escape route and not to be trapped. It would also serve to drive the surviving ancestors out from their ancient home to find a new home.

Claustrophobia reflects itself in numerous ways in human behaviour. Clearly there is claustrophobia if you crawl down a pothole; however the fear of tight spaces is evident in much more common things. The main effects of this are incorporated in our buildings. We build rooms to a certain size. If the ceilings are too low that induces a sense of claustrophobia. If the rooms are too small that induces a sense of claustrophobia. We need clear exits in our rooms with doors we can see. This behaviour all stems from evolution and comes from the time our rock crevice home was a trap.

A fascinating fear I believe we need to understand in order to understand human evolution is the fear of the dark. This fear is deeply engrained in the human psychology and has caused me untold torment in finding an explanation. I have moved it around in time to try and find where it fits. It should be born in mind that I am looking for evolutionary purpose to this fear. This means that it served a purpose and those that developed the fear had a better chance of survival. It also needs to be born in mind that this fear is not a simple fear of the night. There is no point in being afraid simply of the night because there is nothing any creature can do about that. Rather the fear serves to modify behaviour in the dark. At this point in evolution it should also be born in mind that we were nocturnal predators and our eyesight would have been much better adapted for night vision. We would have seen in black and white. There were no cones in the eye only rods. Rods are much more sensitive to light and dark and evolved to detect movement. In the modern human eye the last vestiges of nocturnal vision are left around the edge of the retina. This part of the eye is made up purely of rods and has not changed because it has not been necessary for the edge of the eye to change. If you try it you will find you can still see at night out the corner of your eye. This is what is left of the ancestor's nocturnal black and white vision.

The characteristics of the fear of the dark in children is a fear of going to sleep with the light out along with an accompanying fear of monsters. The combination of these two characteristics comes from our crevice home and the traumatic events we faced there. We were attacked and killed in our beds. These attacks actually took place in the day when we slept however it was pitch black in the depths of the crevice. We evolved so that we slept away from the depths nearer to the entrance where we could still see. Should anything disturb our slumbers we could see the danger and stand a better chance of escape. I imagine we were fairly light sleepers and needed to be. The fears we developed at this time had such an impact it would take us from night into day and from under the ground to over the ground. The fears we evolved caused one of the significant milestones in evolution. The question is what was the creature that created fear of tight spaces, fear of the dark and was itself a monster? The creature was a snake.

The snake is a special creature in the human mind. It has a mythological status, which has arisen out of fear. The snake or serpent is quite often intertwined with the dragon. These are however actually two separate creatures in reality that have become intertwined in mythological story telling.

One such mythological story is that of "The Lambton Worm". John Lambton was fishing one day when he caught a three feet long serpent-like creature with a dragon's head. Repelled by the creature he threw it into a well. However before he did this he looked into the evil creatures eyes and saw himself as a person who had done many wrongs. He decided eventually to redeem himself and travelled to the Holy Lands. Whilst he was away the Lambton Worm grew so huge it could wrap itself nine times around a hill. It killed cows, chickens and people. John Lambton returned home to find out what had happened in his absence. He decided to consult a witch to find out how to destroy the monster. She told him to wear a suit of armour with blades on its surface. However he must also kill the next living thing that he saw after killing the monster or the Lambton's would be cursed for nine generations with no heir dying at home. This doesn't seem a particularly nasty curse to me. Anyway John Lambton donned a suit of armour with blades sticking out of it and fought the creature. When it wrapped itself around him it was sliced into pieces and died. The next living creature he saw was his father. Being a nice chap he didn't kill his father but his favourite dog instead, which wasn't so nice. The trick didn't work and the curse took effect with the Lambtons not dying at home for a long time.

The significance of the myth is obviously in the description of the monster as a snake-like creature and the corresponding association with evil. There are many other myths involving snakes. There is Medusa, an evil Gorgon from Greek mythology with hair of snakes. Again from Greek mythology we have Hydra, a snake monster with nine heads. In Norse mythology there is the "Midgard Serpent", a giant serpent that circled the Midgard world. In Egyptian myth there is Apepi, another giant serpent on which bad weather was blamed. In general the snake is associated with evil; however there is also respect for this ancient adversary.

The snake is associated with cleverness as well as evil and this association is illustrated in the Bible. Genesis chapter 3 records "Now the serpent was more subtil than any beast of the field which the Lord God had made." The Bible goes on to further record the snake becoming a cursed creature "And the Lord God said unto the serpent, because thou hast done this, thou art cursed above all cattle, and every beast of the field. Upon thy belly shalt thou go, and dust shalt thou eat all the days of thy life". These passages are from the fall of Adam and Eve from the Garden of Eden and there is shall we say an entanglement with the old one-eyed snake.

The snake has significance far above the creature we see today. True it is dangerous but it doesn't account for that many human deaths now. There are numerous other creatures such as lions, tigers, crocodiles and mosquitoes that are quite dangerous but are not associated with evil in the same way. The snake's significance I believe comes from this point in evolution. It inflicted sustained and substantial traumatic losses on the ancestor in his crevice home. The snakes association with evil arose out its successful predation on the human ancestor and we have inherited the memory of the trauma it inflicted on us. The fear of this creature comes from evolution and is not an imaginary fear born out of ignorance but a real fear that forms part of the mind we have inherited from our millionth or whatever great grandparents. It can be noted that there is no comic book superhero called snake man. We remember too well what the snake did to us.

The fears of the dark and tight spaces and monster snakes would drive us from our crevice home out into the open. There was an ability that we had developed in our rocky environment that would lead us to our new home. It was here that we had developed the ability to climb. Now however it would not be rocks that we would climb but trees.

Chapter Seven

Utopia in the trees

Life in the trees was relatively safe. Our greatest foe the snake would evolve his behaviour in pursuit of us and eventually evolved into the tree snake. However his evolution was slower than ours and he didn't change his physical form substantially. We would evolve more quickly both physically as well as mentally in the progression towards our current primate form.

The food the ancestor had previously eaten was not so abundant in the trees. There was a food source though that was even easier to catch with the right physical characteristics and this was fruit. Substantial changes would occur to the body through natural selection. Firstly there was a change from a nocturnal existence to a daylight existence. This was a necessary change for the ability to see clearly was essential for a life in the trees. Lack of vision in this environment would lead to the risk of falling and danger of serious injury particularly as we gradually evolved to be larger in size. One of the most important physical changes occurred to the eye.

Because the new food was fruit and fruit doesn't tend to run around, it was not movement that was necessary for vision but colour. The eye would need to develop colour vision to be able to pick out fruit. The centre of the eye evolved and rods changed into cones as a matter of necessity. Cones are the light receptors that distinguish colour. The cone splits the light and detects different wavelengths hence colour. The very centre of the eye is made up purely of cones and it was this part of the eye that was used to find the new source of food.

The light that is the brightest to the human eye is that which falls in the spectrum as a yellowish green. It was this colour that the eye needed to distinguish, as this was the colour of fruit and leaves. The eye however now had a hybrid character, being adapted to finding fruit but also retaining the characteristics of a predator. The nocturnal predator characteristics were now diluted to the extent that the eye only really retained a defensive capacity at night with periphery nocturnal vision.

The other physical changes that were necessary for survival were an improved ability to climb in trees. Tree climbing involved the need for reach to collect fruit. Arms and legs correspondingly grew longer. The ancestor's body developed these physical changes and it was those that did that survived. Hands and fingers developed from paws for improved grip on branches and fruit. Jaws became shorter and teeth developed from slicing incisors to chewing molars. In the trees we became the kind of physical form that we recognise in our selves today. This form is that of a primate.

With fruit being the new source of food, man's ancestor tastes changed and he developed a sweet tooth and liked this new food. We have inherited this sweet tooth. We add sugar to many of our foods and drinks. Virtually all children like sweets and this desire comes from this point in evolution when sugary fruit formed our diet. The ancestor made the canopy of the forest his permanent home. In this niche he would eventually become supreme; however he would not forget his previous existence because it was etched in his mind for all time. In a future time some of his past experience would serve him again. He would remember his previous carnivorous diet and in time it would serve to be the diet that created modern human evolution.

Our diet of fruit meant that we did not evolve into natural born killers of higher life forms. At the time we ascended the trees we were small mouse sized creatures that ate bugs and worms. At the time of our descent from the trees in a time to come we would be much larger creatures that ate bananas. Through all this time we evolved as fruit eaters, which would mean we would never naturally enjoy killing animals. Perhaps our earlier evolution of being the hunted would mean we even evolved a natural aversion against killing. We know what it is like being killed. I have felt the guilt of killing, having taken my lambs to slaughter. We kill through necessity not because we like it.

The ancestor of man had an easy existence in the forest with a plentiful supply of fruit. There was no need for hard work or effort because the forest provided everything. This was an idyllic time. There were only a few natural predators in the trees and they were not too difficult to avoid. He was a lazy creature because there was no need for effort. He could indulge in pleasure because that was all he needed to do. This time in evolution was the only time that man or his ancestors lived a near perfect existence for which he was physically suited. In the future we would always struggle in a world for which we were not physically adapted. This time and place was the first Garden of Eden as portrayed in the Bible.

Pleasure seeking took two simple forms. One of the pleasures was eating the other was sex. The females didn't need the males for rearing the young because of the easy food source. There were no seasons in the forest as it was close to the equator. The female reproductive cycle was all year round as food was abundant all year round. Sexual behaviour was very promiscuous with females and males frequently mating with as many partners as they fancied. There would have been no real cooperative social structure as such at this time for there would have been no need for one. There was group living but not in any especially organised fashion. There would simply be animal based behaviour, which basically took the form of a free for all. This was a time of plenty in all respects and formed a significant layer of human behaviour.

The characteristics we inherited from this period in evolution are observable today and are distinct from the earlier fear driven core of the human mind. This period of safety and assured survival gave the opportunity for these characteristics to develop.

Humans today have a desire for pleasure and this desire comes from this pleasurable original existence. The pursuit of pleasure is a fundamental driving force behind human behaviour. Pleasure seeking takes the form of sexual activity beyond the point of functionality. There is the taking of pleasure inducing substances such as alcohol, tobacco and certain less legal materials. These things are all taken to try and get to a pleasurable utopia for it is from this utopia we came. Pleasure seeking is a function of the mind above and beyond basic animal function. It is observable in other primates with chimps indulging in excess sexual activity above and beyond the point of functionality.

There is also an underlying laziness in the human character. This is represented in many ways in the modern world. Commercial inventions, businesses and technology are frequently designed with the purpose of making life easier. We have cars because driving is easier than walking. There are automatic washing machines, microwaves, ready meals and Chinese takeaways. All these things are based on making existence easier and this all goes back to an underlying laziness in the human character. Some people try to reject this part of human nature but there is no point in my view. Laziness makes us who we are. This desire all comes from a utopian existence at this point in evolution.

Promiscuous sexual behaviour is one of the fundamental driving forces behind human sexuality. Both male and female evolved to take greater pleasure in the sex act. It would take a little longer than it used to. There was a limit however on the length of time that sex would take and this was brought about by the very fact we were promiscuous. We had our quota to get through and so we couldn't hang around for too long. This is observable in the male mind

42

today. Premature ejaculation is not actually premature at all but rather a basic sexual program from early sexual behaviour. This type of behaviour is very much animal based. Where there is volume to sexual encounters the sexual act is quick. This is observable in herd animals where there is a single dominant male with many females. Basic sexual response is a core and ancient part of human programming, which hasn't fundamentally changed from early evolution. This behaviour has however been modified by subsequent layers of later evolutionary programming.

The females were attracted by a certain characteristic in the males and that characteristic was physical size. The taller males had longer reach and evolutionary advantage in accessing food. This is observable today. Women tend to be attracted by taller men and this stems from the time it served the evolutionary advantage of improved reach. When we think of later evolution we find that tallness doesn't really serve any especial evolutionary benefit. It is reaching for fruit where it serves benefit. We find that this period produced female domination of sexual behaviour, which has survived to this day. In times of plenty women take control as they are able to rear children on their own.

The lifestyle in the trees meant that the attractiveness of size to the female and plenty of food complimented each other. Not only did this primate indulge to excess in the mating area but he also indulged to excess in the eating department. It was to be this greed for food that would prove to be man's ancestor's downfall from the idyllic existence. Never again would life be the same and it all came about through one of the frailties that the human mind has inherited. This frailty would become hated and thought of as a sin. This hatred all stems from this original time. Greed was to be the ancestor's downfall.

Greed for food is an inherited problem in Western societies today. Food is plentiful and we can eat as much as we like. We continue to grow larger; however this is mainly in the outward direction rather than the upward direction. High levels of obesity occur and the human mind fights a constant battle with the guilt of it. This all stems from this beginning and the future torment that man would endure because of his frailty of greed.

The Bible records the same version of events that I describe but in an abstract way. The reasons for the Biblical downfall of Adam and Eve and their expulsion from the Garden of Eden are recorded in Genesis chapter 2.

16. And the Lord God commanded the man, saying, of every tree of the garden thou mayest freely eat:
17. But of the tree of knowledge of good and evil , thou shalt not eat of it : for in the day that thou eatest thereof thou shalt surely die.

The references in these two passages are about greed. It can be interpreted that this greed is greed for food if the trees are thought of literally as fruit trees. Alternatively the desire for knowledge can be thought of as greed. There were plenty of trees to eat from apart from the tree of knowledge. These early passages are all about greed because it was greed that was the fundamental reason for mankind's ancestors descending from the trees.

Over time the ancestor of man grew larger and larger on the plentiful supply of fruit in the forest. As he grew larger behaviour changed. Instead of staying day and night in the trees he descended from the trees at night to sleep on the forest floor. He now needed to be fully conscious in the tree top environment. Those ancestors that did fall asleep high in the canopy would increasingly literally fall out of bed to their deaths. It is from this point in evolution that the very expression "fall out of bed" originates. When children fall out of bed today they might experience a descent of a foot or two although it still hurts. Then the descent would have been perhaps fifty feet or maybe more if you can imagine that. This was the start of our descent from the trees.

By this time man's ancestor was much larger than at the time of his ascent of the trees. The adults would learn that there was nothing now to be afraid of on the ground. The forest predators were not huge anymore. They were only a similar size to man's ancestor. Not only did this serve to protect the ancestor but also his absence from the ground protected him. He was new to the forest floor and wasn't the sort of prey any of the predators had developed a taste for eating. The children however still had natural behaviour until the learnt behaviour took over. They were still fearful of the ground in the dark. And so began the bedtime routine of extracting the children from the trees at dusk so as to get them asleep before night fell. We still go through this routine every night with our own children. It can be just as exasperating now as it was then. Now we tend to have to take them back up the stairs to bed rather than having to go up the tree to bring them down as we did then.

One of the most significant associations we make with hominoid species is the ability to stand upright and walk on two legs. I however view this ability in a different light to convention and why is that not surprising? Rather than this ability actually being initially developed on the ground I believe it was developed in the trees. Our clever ability at balancing on our back legs helped us stand on lower branches and reach into the canopy for food. Unfortunately we weren't quite as clever or as good at balancing as we thought we were. This ability only helped us fall off the tree. I believe we could already stand upright by the time we took to the ground.

We continued to grow to the point where we were too large to climb in the canopy of the forest. Our ancestor found moving through the trees quite difficult and actually suffered more falls than his other primate relatives. We didn't like being high in the trees. The branches couldn't support our weight. Through natural selection we developed a fear that would drive us from our home. We developed the fear of heights.

Fear of heights is a basic human fear that many people have. This fear is a very important clue and plays a significant role in establishing human evolution. It hasn't simply appeared out of nowhere but performed an evolutionary function that comes from our primeval past. I believe this fear affected all hominoid species and was the very foundation and starting point for hominoid development.

At this time quite clearly there were only naturally occurring features. The only high features were cliffs and trees. Our previous existence in the rocks was not the place we developed this fear for if it had been we would not have taken to living in the trees. With humans being primates and primates live in trees this fear can only realistically come from trees. This conclusion is the only logical conclusion for the fear of heights. The way our ancestor became scared of heights is by seeing his fellow beings fall and die.

I wonder how many of us have had the dream that I have had. This dream is one of falling but never actually reaching the ground. I believe this dream is from our time in the trees. Fear of heights would become etched on the mind and through natural selection the ancestors that were scared of heights descended from life in the canopy of the forest and started living on the forest floor.

There is an interesting difference between fear of heights and fear of the dark. This difference is that fear of the dark generally disappears in adult hood but fear of heights generally doesn't. The reason for this is that we have lots of experience of the dark and learnt behaviour eventually overrides natural behaviour once we learn there is nothing to be afraid of. As far as heights are concerned we do not generally have experience of heights at all and do not learn not to be afraid of them. The few people that do experience heights do learn not to be afraid of them unless they fall off. By then it's a bit late to learn to be afraid again.

Chapter Eight

Our evolution as a hominoid species

Life on the forest floor was different to the canopy in so far as the source of food was different. Much of the fruit the ancestor had once eaten was now out of reach. Alternative food had to be found. It would be now that intelligence started to develop along with physical changes that arose out of a matter of necessity.

One of the earliest hominoid finds was made in the Middle Awash region of Aramis, Ethiopia. This creature was a large ape and dates from 4.4 million years ago. The remains that have been found include teeth, cranial and post cranial fragments of over 50 individuals, which were preserved in strata of fossilised wood, with remnants of Columbine Monkeys. Savannah-associated fauna proved to be rare in the strata, which supports the view that the first hominoids lived on the forest floor. This is the transition that would logically be expected.

The fossils show that this hominoid had front teeth that were regularly used for clamping and pulling. I believe that there is a pretty good chance that we had started to eat some meat as well as vegetation. If you have ever tried eating just leaves I think you will agree it doesn't form a very tasty diet. The transition from the canopy of the forest to living on a substantially meat based diet on the savannah would be a gradual process that arose out of necessity as the environment changed. Looking at the numbers of individuals found in the Aramis find it is likely that there would significant pressure to find sufficient food. This pressure would lead to rapid evolutionary progress in hominoid natural selection.

Archaeological finds at Lake Turkana in Kenya have established further clues on hominoid evolution. This hominoid discovery dated at around 4 million years old is identified with larger canine teeth with stronger and larger molar teeth than the 4.4 million year old find. The dental evidence tends to suggest increased carnivorous as well as herbivorous physical adaptation. The significance of this is that it suggests that food availability in the forest was not in balance with hominoid needs. This hominoid physically evolved to access a wider food supply both in terms of killing ability of the jaw but also in grinding ability of vegetation.

Footprints, teeth and jawbone remains from two-dozen hominoids have been found on the shore of an ancient lake at Laetoli in Tanzania. The finds have been dated at 3.6 million years old. Further finds have been discovered at Lake Turkana in Kenya with the skeleton of a female dating from 2.9 million years ago. This archaeological evidence provides useful clues as to the physical characteristics and the location of habitat of these hominoids. The remains have shown that this ancestor had a large jaw. There is also an observed significant difference in size between the male and female. Males were estimated to be around 1..5 meters high with females around 1.1 meters tall. This size difference ties in with the reason for the hominoid decent from the trees that being an increase in size accentuated by male attractiveness being linked to size. It is however the location of the finds that is most significant and that location is at the lakeside.

The ancestors chose to live by the waters edge for two reasons. Firstly we required water. Our digestive system had adapted to a fruit diet and we required relatively high amounts of fluid. Secondly the ancestor's prey would need to come to water sources to drink. It would be at this time that the prey would be most vulnerable to attack from the ancestors. Half the potential escape route would be blocked by water on a straight shore. On a peninsular even greater than half the escape route would be blocked. Out on open plain or in the forest a full 360 degrees escape route would be available. Therefore it was by the waters edge that the ancestors would live and wait for the prey.

The question is how did the ancestors kill their prey? Firstly there was biting. Archaeological remains show strong jaws and an increase in canine size in the hominoid find from 4 million years ago compared to the older 4.4 million year old find. This method of killing would only be effective on relatively small animals. By this point in evolution physical adaptation had reached its limit for the ancestor. No longer would increasing jaw size be sufficient for survival. The primate anatomy was not capable of adapting further to become a better predator. It would be mental adaptation that took over from here. You try biting a sheep or cow to death not to be recommended I think.

To kill larger prey an alternative would be needed. Archaeological discoveries of hominoid remains 2.5 million years old have shown an increase in brain size compared to the 3.6-2.9 million year old finds. Additionally there is a reduction in the size of canine teeth and the face is more vertical. These characteristics suggest a move away from killing with the jaw to a more intelligent method of killing. This new method involved the first use of tools.

In the 1950's an archaeological find was made in South Africa at Makapansgat. The find was estimated to be 3-4 million years old. The remains were a pile of canine bones that appeared to be stockpiled as tools. This discovery suggests significant pressure on hominoids with migration and adaptation. The question is how did we evolve to kill larger animals?

The ancestor observed the way the supreme predators killed and tried to copy them. To do this he collected the predators own killing tools and these were their jaws. He used these tools for killing; however he learned a technique of his own based on observation of the way big cats killed. They killed by biting the throat of prey and causing strangulation. The ancestor killed at the same place however he cut the throat with his canine jaw tool. This tool was the first handsaw. It would be from this basic tool that future tool development would evolve. We still use the handsaw today and its design is based on the observation of the jaw.

Over time the environment cooled and this cooling lead to the forests receding in favour of savannah as rainfall declined. Climate studies have shown a cooling of the climate in Africa from around 3 million to 2.4 million years ago. Areas that were once forest were now grasslands. The consequence of this environmental change was an increase in the size of animals. By looking at Africa today we get an idea of the size of animal that occupies savannah and grassland environments. These animals range in general size from gazelle up to elephants. Forest dwelling animals by contrast tend to be smaller because there is less space to move around in. There is also evolutionary advantage in a larger size as protection from predators. The larger you are the safer you are.

The increase in size of the ancestor's prey lead to a change in the killing tool he used, forced out of necessity. 2.4 million years ago man's ancestor made the oldest stone tools that have ever been found. Considering the changes in the environment and the types of herbivores that had now evolved it does seem logical that it would be around this time that a change in killing tool would happen.

The oldest stone tools that are known of are called the Oldowan tools and were located in the Gona and Omo Basins in Ethiopia. The previous killing tool, the saw, had substantial limitations. The main limitation was the depth of cut. The second limitation was that the teeth had a habit of falling out. It was however these teeth that would give rise to the blue print for a killing tool that would evolve eventually all the way into the sword. The ancestor used observation and ingenuity to develop his new killing tool. This tool was the legendry hand axe. It wasn't however designed by chance but was a copy of a naturally occurring tool. This tool was used for the same killing purpose and it was the tooth.

The ancestor learned by observation and he observed one of the teeth that had fallen out of his canine jaw saw. He would have by now realised that it was the incisor teeth that were the teeth that cut. The canine teeth were fearsome looking. They were not however the teeth that did the cutting work. He used the incisor tooth as the blueprint for his tool and with his ingenuity crafted a scaled up version out of stone. He created the hand axe. The logic he used was simple. The larger the tooth he had the larger animals he could kill. This may seem simplistic today however archaeological finds do confirm this thought process. Later stone hand axes dated at around 1.5 million years old show how the hand axe developed over this million-year period. These later hand axes called Acheulean tools are crafted to be much closer copies of incisor teeth. They are sharper than the earlier tools and much larger.

Not all the innovation in the development of the later hand axes was actually practical. By copying incisor teeth more accurately the holding end was made sharp. By making them larger they were much more difficult to use. The logic that created the hand axe was however to create the perfect tooth and make it as large as possible. Modern human behaviour is the same. "The bigger the better." 4X4's take over the Chelsea streets on the school run. Small cars would make logical sense as they are cheaper to run, easier to park and safer to pedestrians. The 4x4 would perhaps be safer in a high-speed accident; however rapid progress and London streets do not really go together. Still, human nature is not perfectly logical and neither was the ancestors mind perfect.

Human nature with regards to design remains the same as the ancestor's nature. The closer something resembles nature the more beauty we see in it. Aeroplanes have been created based on the observation of birds. The Spitfire is more beautiful than a modern jet because it looks more like a bird. It is this logic and appreciation of beauty that drove the development of the hand axe.

We still kill in the same way today as we killed with our hand axes two million years ago with throat cutting remaining the basic method of slaughter. This method has remained the same for such a long period of time because it was effective in the beginning. The hand axe was such a common tool because it was such an important tool. It was the tool that fed the ancestor.

The ancestor of man was a hunter but the question is did he become the hunted? He was clearly in no position to physically defend himself against the large cats that were the supreme predators at this time. Would you like to fight a lion with a hand axe? I don't think so. It was by fate of evolution that our ancestor did not become a staple source of food for the supreme predators. He had been in the trees when they were evolving their tastes on the forest floor. They didn't recognise him or know what he was. By looking at Africa today we get an idea of just how the big cats preferences for food are expressed.

Big cats prefer to hunt herd animals. Humans are killed but they are not their staple source of food. Big cats have an inbuilt instinct for hunting certain game. Cheetahs like gazelle because they are solitary hunters and this is the size of animal it can safely hunt on its own. Lions tackle larger game such as buffalo as they hunt in prides. They cooperate together and are able to bring down the larger animals. They can afford to take more risks because if one gets injured its offspring at least has a chance of getting food from the kill of others in the pride.

The predators about at this time didn't particularly take that much notice of the ancestor if he kept out of their way. He was an alien entity to them. The size of animal the ancestor preyed on meant he only really needed to come close to the solitary big cats. He killed animals of a similar size to a gazelle. Bison sized creatures were generally too large to kill safely with a hand axe. These animals would not become prey until the advent of the spear although relatives of man would take up the challenge. The ancestor developed a relatively stable and safe way of life based on a carnivorous diet.

At the time of the first tools 2.4 million years ago the ancestors mainly survived through sheer effort. Despite tools they still lived in a hostile environment and were not physically well adapted. The quickest organ to adapt and change was the brain. Substantial physical changes would have taken much longer to turn a primate into a well-adapted predator or herbivore. This would have taken millennia of time and probably could never have happened. I consider it would be inconceivable for the human digestive system to change to become like a cow with four stomachs in such a short evolutionary time scale. Equally to change into a dog or big cat would be inconceivable. The only organ available for substantive change in such a short period of time was the brain and that is what did change as a matter of necessity.

Catching gazelle type animals sounds fairly difficult to us today especially bearing in mind that there were no spears or bows and arrows at this time. However we need to consider this. Just the same as hominoids were not recognised as prey neither were they recognised as predators. They could get close to the creatures of the day provided they didn't make sudden movements. I look at the way my chickens behave with my cats. They are not scared of them because they have no evolutionary experience of the domestic cat. Equally the domestic cat doesn't see the chicken as prey because it has no evolutionary experience of the chicken. The same would have been the case for hominoids. They would not be recognised to start with and it is only through the process of evolution that animals became scared of them. This process takes a while. It is quite interesting to note that cows are afraid of sticks. Now a stick by its self is not particularly dangerous. However a stick in the form of a spear is. Has the cow evolved to fear spears? It could have.

Having made the above point catching prey did get harder. Through natural selection the digestive systems of these animals developed so that they did not need to come to the lakes and rivers to drink as frequently. This forced evolutionary change in the ancestor. He now had to start travelling from the lakes and rivers to where these animals grazed. The need for travelling meant changes to the body to create it into a better walker.

By around 2 million years ago the ancestor had developed longer legs and an increased brain size. He had also grown in stature, which would suggest that the diet he lived on was reasonably plentiful in supply. Mental and some social ability would be necessary to catch his prey. It is likely although not certain that he worked in small groups and developed a way of herding animals so that they could get close enough to catch and kill the animals.

With social cooperation in hunting comes the need for communication. There has been much debate over when language first originated. My view is that this was much later. The method of communication most suited to hunting is the use of gesticulation. The shouting of instructions when sneaking up on prey rather gives the game away. In modern day battles gesticulation is used to issue instructions in order that a soldier doesn't give away his position. The same would be true in this early prehistoric hunt.

This hominoid ancestor was a successful hunter and his numbers increased. There was however only enough space for a certain number in the old central areas and the excess numbers would be forced to migrate. This migration would have been through pressure of competition. The most successful and competitive hominoids held the central old territories. The less competitive hominoids were the ones that moved. Migration occurred into North Africa and Eastern Asia. Competition would be based on aggression with battles between hominoid gangs. Fights would break out over hunting grounds. The ancestors of the first Homo sapiens were one of the most competitive hominoids at this time. Our migration out of Africa was the last hominoid migration.

The increase in hand axe sizes with the rise of the Acheulean tool industry does suggest that from 1.5 million years ago hominoids were moving to kill larger animals. Larger animals required larger teeth to kill them at least this was the wisdom of the day. Hominoid remains dated at 0.8 million years old show how the ancestor physically changed. Body size increased along with brain size. Interestingly the finds of this hominoid have been found with dismembered and burned hominoid remains. This suggests that there was significant pressure for survival. The tendencies that would drive evolution on to form modern man were showing themselves. This evolution would be dominated by competition between hominoids. The world would become a more aggressive and brutal place from now on.

Chapter Nine

The move to modern man

And so we begin our progression towards the single-family existence. By fate of evolution the ancestors of man became a little bit quicker runners than their contemporaries that they lived with. This gave competitive advantage. This advantage was not in relation to the animals they hunted for they were and always would be much quicker than the hominoids that hunted them. Four legs are quicker than two. The advantage was over the other hominoids they hunted with. We could get to the hunting grounds quicker than our relatives. This difference would be the start of a rift that would see the creation of man.

The ancestor of man continued hunting gazelle sized animals. The hominoids he had hunted with started to hunt larger game as competition for prey intensified. The key to big game hunting lay with improved social skills. No longer could a single hominoid hold an animal and kill it. These larger animals required the cooperation of several men to hold and kill the animal. This improvement in social cooperation would in time serve to give these hominoids superiority over the ancestors of the first men.

The size of prey is a key to evolution. It is by observing domestic farm animals that I have reached this conclusion. It is possible for a single man to hold and kill a sheep with a hand axe. It is not possible for a single man to hold and kill a cow with a hand axe. Cows are extremely strong with thick hides and the cow's ancestor is likely to have been significantly wilder than its domesticated descendant. Today cows are not especially compliant and even getting a needle through a cow's hide let alone a hand axe is pretty difficult. Through dealing with domesticated farm animals you realise just how hard the practicalities of killing were for the ancestors. It would require the sheer brute force of a substantial number of hominoids to over power and kill a cow-sized creature with just hand tools.

The very thing that had given the ancestors of man competitive advantage would now come back to haunt them. They had used running rather than improved social abilities to survive. The improved social abilities were however the facets that would make what were now relatives of man the dominant force that held the central areas. The ancestor of man now developed running not to gain competitive advantage in the hunt but to save his own life. He would come to be the hunted and he had to run for his life.

The climate continued to become harsher and competition for land in the valley became fiercer between the hominoids there. This pressure would result in the grim evolution of hominoid behaviour towards greater cannibalism. Remains of hominoid fossils are increasingly associated with dismembered and burnt hominoid remains as evolution progressed. This behaviour served two purposes. Firstly there was the eating of hominoids for food. Secondly there was the fear element induced in the hominoids that found they were being eaten. This fear would serve to push them away from the hunting grounds that were already under pressure from over hunting.

The size of the groups that man's ancestor lived in shrank under pressure of competition. Other hominoid groups started to become more successful through improvements in their cooperative behaviour. These groups became more aggressive towards the ancestors of the first Homo sapiens. We struggled to survive in ever shrinking numbers and this in turn led to a cycle of decline. The smaller the groups got the less sociable the ancestors evolved to be. We are progressing towards a single-family existence. Man was not in fact a sociable creature at all when he was created in the form we recognise as ourselves. People still exist today that have this original mind function to show this to be the case. This is what is being observed in the autistic personality.

The shores of the lakes and the edges of the rivers were becoming increasingly more dangerous places to live. The ancestors were now out numbered in the groups they lived in and would lose the fights that broke out with the other groups of relative hominoids. Through losing fights this would lead to a shift in the behaviour of the ancestors of man. This shift was to avoid fighting by running away. The next human fear was born and that was the fear of relative hominoid species.

Remains of what are thought to be man's closest ancestor were found in 1993 near a village called Herto in Ethiopia. The remains consisted of two men and a six or seven year old child and are dated at around 160,000 years old. The characteristics of the skull suggest these men were larger than modern humans but in other respects fairly similar. These skulls were found to have cut marks on them, which suggested that the bodies had their flesh, removed. There is a vein of thought that thinks this may have been some ritualistic burial practice. I feel it is much more likely that these men were killed. The fear of relative hominoid species was realised with grim effect on the day these men died. Normally they could have run away however this day they had a child with them and either had to leave the child or stand and fight. They chose not to run and I suspect faced one of the worst deaths in the hands of relative hominoid gangs. These men were skinned alive. It was events like these that reinforced the fear and hatred of relative hominoid species. It would force the evolution of the first true human beings.

Fear of relative hominoid species is evident in children and in adults today. In children this fear takes the form of what we call "fear of the bogie man". This man that children are scared of is like a human but is not human. This bogie man came to get children and the reason for this fear is because that is what the bogie man did. He was real at this time and the fear of him would never be forgotten.

In adults fear of relative hominoid species is realised in a fear of the closest sized primate to man. This primate is the gorilla. People dress up in gorilla suits to create entertainment through fear. The escaping gorilla forms entertainment in fairground attractions. In the autumn the Goose Fair would come to Nottingham and on occasion I would go into the Ape-man sideshow. The Ape-man, who was in fact only a man dressed up in a gorilla suit, would escape from his cage and cause panic in the audience. This show is based on the fear of relative hominoid species and the entertainment plays on that fear. Everybody knows that the Ape-man isn't real but the basic fear instinct overrides that conscious knowledge and creates the entertainment. Films and television programs have been made to create entertainment based on this fear. An early film on this subject, which created a big impact in its time, was King Kong. In the film the Gorilla was created into a monster. We all know that gorillas are not monsters however the film played on the basic human fear of hominoid species and that is the reason it achieved the success it did. In more recent years the fear has been exploited in the television series and films about the Planet of the Apes. This entertainment centred on human inferiority to another hominoid species and proved popular and scary at the time it was made. This was because it was based on reality although we perhaps didn't realise it.

Running away from other hominoids worked for adults because of their running ability. They were able to out run the groups of relative hominoids that came after them. It was a different matter for the children however. They were vulnerable to attack. The children could not run fast enough to escape. They resorted to an ancient instinct and that instinct was to hide.

Childhood games give us clues to the evolution of human behaviour. These games are inherited and have created entertainment for the countless generations of children. The games however were not for entertainment in the beginning. These games were the method through which natural selection took place. It was the children that were good at hiding that survived. They passed this ability on to their children and that ability was established through an interest in it.

The interest in hiding has been inherited to this day and is shown in the childhood game called "Hide and Seek". The feature of this game is that the child who is selected to be on has to hunt the the other children who hide. There is a natural desire to be the hunted. The game shows that man was not the hunter but was the hunted. Had the opposite been true with man being the hunter then Hide and Seek would take a different form. The child that is selected as being on would be the one that hides, with the rest trying to find him. This is not how the game is played.

Another childhood game that comes from natural selection at this point in evolution is a game called Tig or Tag. The feature of this game is to run away from the child that is selected as being on. Again the natural position to take in the game is the one who is chased. One child has to be forced to run after the others by being picked. Had man been the chaser in evolution then the game would take the form of the child that is picked being the chased and this is not the case. Children naturally desire to run away and this serves to develop their skills of evasion. It was these skills that were necessary in adulthood for survival. It was those ancestors that developed the skills that survived and in turn passed them on to their children. Children would practice and practice these games and they formed the basis of human behaviour at this time. The children that didn't develop such interests would find themselves as dinner for the bogie man.

This lifestyle of fear served to affect the behaviour of the ancestor of man in terms of where he chose to live. Fear would serve to force him to start to migrate away from the lakes and rivers. He would start to move to places that were less conjested and safer. These locations would be within walking distance of the rivers and lakes to start with. The small group of ancestors would walk to water each day to drink. Gradually through competition this walk would get longer as the ancestors were pressed further out away from the original central areas.

Natural selection would serve to select the children with the best travelling abilities. It would be these children that would survive to pass these characteristics on to their children. Legs would become longer and bodies lighter. The groups shrank in size as only the best adapted survived. Brains would grow larger through the natural selection of intelligence for survival.

Increased intelligence became a neccessity now to find food and avoid capture. Operating in shrinking numbers man's ancestor found it increasingly difficult to catch gazelle type creatures. This animal was diminishing in number. Smaller and more diverse animals were caught. With this a variety of techniques were needed which lead to increasing intelligence. It was the very requirement of being a hunter accessing a range of food sources as well being the hunted that forced human intelligence beyond that of the superior hominoids at this time. Only those that evolved survived. Gradually through time the modern human body and basic mind was formed.

The process of retreat continued until eventually this retreat ended up in the mountains around the Rift Valley. It was here that behaviour changed again. It would be in this place that women and children would stay and man would travel alone. There was one of the necessities of life in the mountains but not the other. There was water but there was no food. Man however was able to carry food but he was not able to carry water. This made the mountains a possible place to live even though it was not sought after because of the lack of food. This place would become home. It was now too far for the whole family to travel together; this place was however safe. The other hominoids did not come here as it was too far for them to bother to travel. The groups of men were by now very small and ranged in size from perhaps three or four males down to the single male with a similar number of females.

The size of groups is predictable from modern human behaviour. Groups of close friends only number around three or four individuals at most and it is from this point in evolution that these close relationships come from. Friendships are not however characterised by a cooperative relationship in a working sense as we think of work today. When friends see too much of each other or work together they have a habit of falling out. Group relationships based on working cooperation were at this point in evolution in the future. Close friendships are life long and this comes from evolution, as these groups were life long groups. They are characterised by the pleasure in being in the company of friends and sharing. This is how I believe we existed at this time in evolution when we shared food with friends.

Clues to the type of environment we lived in when the modern human mind was being formed in evolution can be found in the types of environment we are naturally attracted to today. These environments form modern day tourist attractions and one of these environments is mountain terrain. There is a natural feeling of safety in the mountains. Mountains are the places people have retreated to in times of crisis. Britons retreated to the Welsh mountains in the face of Saxon invasion in the Dark ages. People climb mountains for recreation and the ascent of Everest is considered one of the greatest human achievements. This desire all comes from evolution when the mountains were home to the closest ancestors of the first men.

Over time the environment became drier and drier. Pressure increased on all hominoids. Only the fastest and cleverest ancestors survived this harsh life of trying to catch food and avoiding the relative hominoid species of man. These first people lived close to the edge of existence and natural selection killed many. This man's brain developed rapidly with this life style.

Chapter Ten

The original clever running men

In the earliest passages of the Bible we find our first reference to man. I am not however going to pretend that I can make evolution fit exactly the Biblical Creation because I can't. The Biblical Creation does however contain elements that do fit with evolution. I consider that the story of Adam and Eve is very close to the truth. It is this appeal to our psychology that draws me to look carefully at the book of Genesis. The argument between creationism and evolution has lasted so long because of the appeal of truth contained in the scriptures. Even the Bible concedes that Adam and Eve were not the first people.

The first human beings are recorded in the Bible in Genesis chapter 1, which reads:

26. And God said, Let us make man in our image, after our likeness: and let them have dominion over the fish of the sea and over the fowl of the air, and over the cattle, and over all the earth, and over every creeping thing that creepeth upon the earth.
27. So God created man in his own image in the image of God created he him. Male and female created he them.
28. And God blessed them and God said unto them "Be fruitful, and multiply, and replenish the earth, and subdue it, and have dominion over the fish of the sea, and over the fowl of the air, and over every living thing that moveth upon the earth.
29. And God said, Behold, I have given you every herb bearing seed, which is upon the face of all the earth, and every tree, in the which is the fruit of a tree yielding seed; to you it shall be for meat.
30. And to every beast of the earth, and to every fowl of the air, and to every thing that creepeth upon the earth,

wherein there is life, I have given every green herb for meat: and it was so.

31. And God saw everything that he had made, and behold, it was very good. And the evening and the morning were the sixth day.

It can be seen from the passages that meat was the source of food in paragraphs 29. and 30. It would seem that the vegetation was for the purposes of creating meat rather than being directly eaten by humans. It can also be seen that there was the concept of sexual freedom in paragraph 28. "Be fruitful, and multiply, and replenish the earth" This statement is in contrast to the latter story involving Adam and Eve where sexual restriction dominates. Most importantly however it can be seen that there is no reference of man communicating with God in the Biblical creation. God is the one doing all the talking. This is because there was no awareness of religious concept at this point in man's evolution. Man had yet to meet God and acquire his soul.

The mountains were home and the first men survived by becoming runners. They ran from the mountains into into the valley floor. It was here they hunted for food which when caught would be carried back home to the mountains. There were two types of running and each had a separate purpose. The first type of running was the sprint and this was for the purpose of escapeing imminent hominoid attack. It wasn't formed out of escaping animal attack or as a hunting technique. Trying to out sprint a lion is completely futile. I havent tried it and don't intend to but believe me I am sure it is. Likewise trying to even out sprint a sheep let alone a gazzel type animal is pretty futile. I have tried this with a sheep and believe me you can't.

The second type of running is long distance running and this was born out of the need to travel. Why run and not walk? The reason for this comes down to the working day. If we take say the maximum distance the modern human can normally run this gives an idea of how a working day may have been. This distance is the length of a marathon. By running man could get to the hunting territory hunt and return home to safety in one day. Had he walked it would have taken him a whole day to get to the hunting territory and back again. Walking at four miles an hour it would have taken approximately six hours to cover the distance of a marathon and another six to get back again. This is twelve hours in total and the whole day. By running this time is cut to six hours travelling time with six hours hunting time. This behaviour of travelling endurance is still part of human behaviour today. Lengthy commutes to work seem to make no sense. However people still do them and this is due to an evolutionary ability to endure travelling long distances to hunting territories. The strong connection people have with home and the safety of where they know overrides the inconvenience of lengthy commuting.

The basic male instinct is to run alone. This is the quickest way to travel. Women can run however most do not run as quickly as men. When children are taken into account then it becomes impossible for a family group to travel in this way. The desire for speed is particularly prevalent in the male mind. Today this takes the form of driving or riding quickly. There is a thrill derived from speed and this thrill forms the basis of the numerous racing activities there are. These activities include running, horse racing and motor sports. The general theme is the faster the better provided you don't fall over, fall off or crash. This desire for speed came from evolution and running.

The balance of risk

At this point I want to look at what I consider to be an important psychological difference between the male and female minds today. This difference regards the differing attitudes towards risk. The female mind is more risk averse than the male mind. The question is where does this difference come from in evolution. Clearly in the trees the risk was the same for everyone. Life by the lake meant similar risks for everyone. For there to be a difference I believe the male and female split up in the activities they undertook. It was the male that undertook the risky activities and the female stayed away from risky situations.

The running man whilst being careful did take calculated risks in order to succeed. He had to come close to relative hominoids and other predators to get close to prey. It was this man's woman that didn't like risks and she stayed in the mountains. When a woman has children she becomes very risk averse and this is a necessary state to be in to ensure the safety of the children. This attitude towards risk kept the children alive. They did not follow the running man to the hunting territories. They stayed at home where the predators and relative hominoids couldn't get them. A woman with children had no chance of escape by running away. Therefore she didn't place herself in a position that meant she ran this risk.

The balance between the male and female minds with regards to risk kept this group alive. The balance of risk occurs between men and women today in the same way as it did at this period in evolution. The female mind remains risk averse when caring for children. I believe the same thing occurred with the clever running man and his woman for a good reason and it came about through natural selection. Only those groups survived where the balance of risk was right.

Coming on to the size of group we can make a logical prediction based on current behaviour, the past and future evolutionary phases along with religious text. We have the group of friends naturally numbering three of four individuals, which comes from the past phase of evolution. The future phase will bring forth the single family, which is what we are progressing towards. In religious text we have the concept of sexual freedom. The logical conclusion therefore is a group of two men along with a similar number of women. This gives us the concept of friendship we recognise today as our "best friend".

Taking the religious concept of sexual freedom we have a number of sexual behaviours that exist today that were formed by this phase of evolution. Firstly we have the desire for a threesome or foursome. This behaviour features quite strongly in pornographic materials and does prove to have sexual appeal. We have the concept of wife swapping which again proves naturally sexually stimulating. In terms of friendship the "best friend" is something all people try to find. This best friend is somebody of the same sex with whom a close bond is formed. This relationship like that of friendship is not characterised by cooperative behaviour in the sense of working together. Best friends have a habit of falling out if they see too much of each other. Everybody has the capacity to have a best friend and whether or not one is found depends rather on luck. At this time in evolution these bonds were easier to establish because the small groups stayed together for life and the children were brought up together. This would in tern establish the bond for the next generation.

The original running man had heightened senses compared to most people today. These senses were closer to the animal world than the modern human world. He could hear his prey sooner. He could see it on the semi arid savannah quicker. He could smell more clearly. When we observe animals we can see that their senses are more acute than our own. It is extremely difficult to sneak up on a sheep they always seem to hear you coming. Dogs have a much more acute sense of smell and hearing than our own. The same was true for us. We used our natural senses to the full in the battle for survival and nature selected for them in full. Further more this man was more sensitive to pain and more careful. He needed to remain uninjured or he could die. There was no society then only your best friend to rely on.

The relative difference in the acuteness of senses is observable today and is identified in the observations of autistic spectrum disorder. Sensitivity to pain can be observed in discomfort with certain types of clothing. Clothes that have prickly textures such as certain types of wool garments can be very difficult for these people to wear. Acute hearing is observable. Irritation can be caused by sounds, which are not normally noticed by most people. In these people there can be heightened vision awareness which means greater detail is observed than would normally be the case. The senses of taste and smell can be more acute with aversion to strong tastes and smells. All these senses served the purpose of survival at this time in human evolution.

This man had another advantage compared with most people today that helped him survive. He had better intuition as to what his prey and predators would do. This intuition developed through natural selection. Those men that could predict how animals would behave had an advantage when hunting. He developed empathy with his prey and understood them. He had closeness with the animal world and this was the only world he knew. This closeness with animals is still seen today and came from evolution. There is a human aversion to animal cruelty and a desire to keep pets.

As we move forward in time the environment becomes harsher and we find that under the pressure of competition the groups of men shrank to the point of a single man. Only the fittest survived and there was no room for compassion. It was a case of "evolve or die". There was no room for the weak and as there would always be a weaker man in a group of two these groups of men split. No longer did people share their food. This was a time of every man for himself and this very saying "every man for himself" is the kind of behaviour that human beings demonstrate in a time of crisis. This was a time of crisis and the single-family existence was born.

In times of crisis we see the core of human behaviour. This behaviour centres on self-preservation. When the thin veil of civilisation breaks down and panic sets in we see our ancient natural instincts at work. These instincts are not directed towards cooperative behaviour. These instincts are very much self focussed born out of self-preservation. Our most basic instinct is that of pure self-preservation. This behaviour comes from early evolution. This is however overridden with latter instincts towards the protection of our children. At the end of this period we see the protection of the family becoming the prime driving force. The family is the basic minimum building block necessary for evolutionary survival and we have inherited this behaviour.

The time of the clever running man was coming to an end. Human intelligence had been created. Now we would see the coming of the most critical period in our evolution. This period would create the original human personality. This personality is the one that is described by Asperger's Syndrome. It was born in a period that saw the human species driven close to extinction.

Chapter Eleven

The single family of one man one woman living in the desert

In my view the single most important characteristic of human behaviour is the single human family. This family is made up of a man a woman and children. This group structure has not occurred by chance. It has been formed by evolution and we are going to look at how humans evolved to live in single families. This is the evolution of monogamy and love.

Love is a peculiar characteristic. Few creatures have the need for it. The ones that do are the ones where both parents are needed to rear young. Some birds pair for life. One sits on the eggs and the other hunts for food. There aren't many creatures however that live like this. The reason is that most creatures haven't found themselves quite as close to the point of extinction as we have been. Both parents would need to be bonded for life to rear children in this time to come. Those people that evolved to love were the ones to survive.

Climate research has established that from around 150,000 to 130,000 years ago Africa underwent a period of arid conditions. I believe it is this period that created the next phase of human evolution. We would become smaller on a more restricted diet in the harsh environment. There would be substantial changes in behaviour that would lead to one of the two core mind types that exist in humans today.

As the environment reached this arid phase the relative hominoids were forced to move to new areas or die. This environment could not support group hunting as the large game had gone. This place was now a virtual desert and with the relative hominoid groups moving away the need for speed reduced. There were no large predators left. Now people walked rather than ran and we create one of the fundamental human activities that is used for recreation today. That recreation is taking a walk. We still like to take a walk in the park and this desire arises from our walking in evolution although it wasn't for recreation then but survival. It is from here that I draw the very title of this book. Shoes are so important to us because of our origin as a walking species. You are now going to stand in those shoes.

Man was so fearful of the relative hominoids that he didn't follow them. We have no evidence so far of Homo sapien migration outside East Africa from as far back in time as this. Man lived in single family groups and in this sized group he had no confidence gained by virtue of numbers. Without confidence the drive to step into the unknown is severly restricted. I believe it was this lack of confidence that prevented human migration at this point. We have a natural strong connection with home and only tend to leave with the confidence that we have some idea of where we are going to. There was no concept of the outside world or what was there. People had survived here for generations before and they remained here. It would be the very fact that man didn't move that would lead to natural selection making him what he would become.

In the desert there were only small animals to live on. This was man's most desperate time and only those men that evolved survived. This was a life dominated by almost constant hunger and was much worse than anything we had previously endured. The original man now lived in a single-family with his wife and children and he started to hunt in a new way. This was a single man and single women working together. No longer was it necessary for a woman to stay in a safe place away from danger because the only risk left was starvation and we couldn't hide from that. This risk could only be avoided by supreme effort on the part of both man and woman. This is the basis of mankind and the original way we lived when we had our hardest and most tormented time in the battle for survival.

By working together man and woman would improve their chance of survival in a very harsh environment where every scrap of food that could be found was needed. This food would have been mainly in the form of reptiles as it is these creatures that are best suited to this environment. Some people still keep reptiles and I believe this fascination comes from an inherited interest in reptiles from the time that is all we had to eat. Genesis chapter 1, refers to man having dominion over "every thing that creepeth the earth." This paragraph refers to reptiles for it is these creatures that "creepeth." Other animals walk, fly or swim. In anything other than the harshest of environments reptiles do not tend to feature as a staple food source. People generally eat cattle, sheep, pigs, chickens, fish, grain, rice or vegetables for the most part. It was reptiles that formed the basis of our diet at this time.

If I were trying to compare this with anything in the world we know today I suppose the closest comparison would be with the Australian Aboriginal existence. Obviously many live in villages nowadays; however we still have knowledge of how they naturally existed in the relatively recent past before we got there and messed it up for them. The Aboriginal life style was based on foraging over a wide area of territory. They caught reptiles to eat and had intimate knowledge of their land with large distances being walked in the hunt for food. This is as close a comparison with the modern world I can make. Even the name Aborigine has an uncanny resemblance to origin as in our original existence.

The consequence of living in a harsh environment gives us reason for an unusual characteristic we have inherited. Humans grow at a much slower pace than most other creatures. In sheep we see rapid growth with sexual maturity reached in just a single year. Cows reach maturity in two and they are much larger than we are. The closest primate in terms of size to us, that being the Gorilla, reaches sexual maturity at about nine years of age. People on the other hand take thirteen of fourteen years to mature. Growth rate is dictated by the amount of food available for conversion into body mass. Having inherited a general size from previous evolution we find a slowing of growth evolves to achieve that general size. Comparing people to Gorillas we could be looking at perhaps a slowing of some 25-30% from previous evolution as a rough estimate. The size itself also evolves to be generally smaller. Along with the slowing of growth comes a slowing of mental maturity in order that the mind and body can remain in harmony. A child with an adult mind doesn't work. It needs to remain in a nurtured state until maturity otherwise we have the concept of the "Tweenager" and I think we know the misery that can inflict.

The balance of present and future

This lifestyle formed the most engrained form of human behaviour of one man and one woman desperately searching for food. They both focussed obsessively. This took slightly different forms. She would be very wide viewing looking everywhere for anything to eat now. He looked and focused obsessively into the future looking for tracks of animals and the food it might lead to. In the modern day this behaviour still exists. I look at my own existence and believe it mirrors how it was for the original man. My wife has a natural desire to come with me when I go out even though I would rather do things alone for the sake of speed. I believe the natural desire not to be left alone means that she wasn't left alone in the original existence. I look into the future to see what may become and my wife looks very much at the present to see what can be done now.

The difference between the male and female minds with regards to present and future is very significant in evolutionary development. It is the balance between the two that is critical for survival and both were and still are needed. The male original mind is not naturally capable of doing both. This mind is very much focussed on a single track. In evolution this was essential for following faint tracks left by animals in the sand with concentration the key. The ability to ignore distraction was important as distraction could lead to tracks being easily lost. At the same time opportunities in the present could not afford to be wasted. It was these opportunities that the female mind was adapted to take advantage of. The female mind when with child is capable of considering several things in quick succession and moving quickly from one track to another. This ability was necessary to be able to look after children along with identifying opportunistic food sources as they arose. This mind was not as concerned with detail for there was no need. Detail was the domain of the male mind. The female mind functioned with less depth but greater width. Only couples with the correct balance of the present and future survived.

We now have the most efficient form of the human decision-making process. This structure survived the hardest time in human evolution and is formed out of a combination of the male and female minds. The male mind provides direction for the future along with the natural ability to accept the risks that the future entails. The female mind naturally operates in the present and provides restraint to the taking of excessive risk. This structure is reflected today in the way a company is run. We have the director providing vision and direction for the future of the company. He works closely with his secretary. The more intimate this relationship is the closer we get to the evolutionary formation of this decision making process. Her function is much more significant however than her title suggests. She provides vision of the present and cautionary restraint to the director and his ambitions for the future. When the two work properly together we have the most efficient, if at times tormented, human decision making team that has ever existed. This torment can be increased somewhat if the director's wife finds out he has been a little too intimate with his secretary.

I have set out the natural balance between male and female. I do have to point out that not all men and not all women seem to have completely typical natural minds. There are some women that behave more men and some men that behave more like women in certain ways. In a similar way to how our sexuality is not completely uniform neither do I believe the male and female thought process to be completely uniform. We do therefore see some women achieving feats that require extraordinary focus and obsession. Likewise we find some men that can achieve extraordinary feats of multi tasking.

Going back to life in the desert the original man developed intuition with his wife. His relationship with her was based on this. Language had not developed at this point in evolution. This was a very simple existence with the obsessive search for food dominating behaviour. This intuition still survives today in couples with original minds. They intuitvely know what each other is doing. My wife has this intuition. She intuitively knows if I am up to something naughty. Mind you that doesn't take much working out. Communication between man and woman in the original life was not extensive nor needed to be with this simple existence. Each had their own work to do and cooperation between the two was all natural. They did not talk and in fact silence was an advantage in this place. Language is only a necessity in a group when dealing with more than one person or asking somebody you don't know intimately for something. The ability to hear the slightest sound could be the difference between eating and not. The lack of a natural understanding of language still shows itself today in people with original minds. Spelling can sometimes seem to be poor. There can be a natural difficulty in remembering names. There were no names in the original existence.

Obsession

This was not a sophisticated man. There was no need for sophistication in this place. This was a simple existence.

Intelligence was not the most essential attribute for survival at this time. There were no relative hominoids or predators to avoid. There were no quick running herbivores to outwit and catch. The most important attribute that kept him and his family alive was focus and obsession. He hunted pretty much all of the time and had to concentrate mentally to compensate for his physical limitations, in order to stay alive. If his other skills failed to yield results he just kept on going. He only stopped when he was successful or when he ran out of energy. He would even hunt when it was dark if he had to. Reptiles would tend to have been inactive at night because they are cold blooded. This would have made hunting easier in some respects. There would have been moonlight to work under, as clouds in this place would have been rare. Man was not adapted for this environment and he struggled desperately in the battle for survival.

Obsession along with intelligence defines us as a species. It is a combination of the two that has given the human race the mental characteristics necessary for domination of the world. Obsession seems to very misunderstood and is almost demonised. It can create problems it is true and does seem a bit odd when the obsession is with something peculiar. The characteristic itself however is essential in genius and is the one characteristic common to all outstanding achievements.

The original innate rules of behaviour

Behaviour would adapt to this harsh environment and only those men and women that evolved survived. Obsession would be the key; however other attributes developed which would play their part in evolution. It was essential to have as large a hunting ground as possible with such a sparse supply of food. This meant that the people alive at this time needed to keep out of each other's way. Too many people in one area would exhaust the meagre food there was. These people would develop another human attribute that would serve an evolutionary purpose for survival and that attribute was shyness. These people became shy of each other.

Shyness is a fundamental human characteristic. This character is reflected in different ways. The original mind in its natural state is introverted and shy. The opposite of this natural state is the extrovert. Both are basically the same however the extrovert has learnt not to be shy. With no natural understanding of interaction with other people extroverts can take their behaviour to the point of becoming very irritating indeed.

Another attribute that developed along with shyness was the concept of personal territory and land ownership. By having personal territory this would serve to prevent conflict between men. Each man had his territory and straying into another man's land could lead to fighting and possibly even death. Boundaries were established and a man would need to survey his territory to ensure boundaries remained in the same place. This behaviour is reflected today. We are naturally a territorial species and mark our boundaries with fences, walls and ditches.

With the concept of ownership of territory came other human attributes that would serve evolutionary purpose for survival. These attributes would in many years to come form the basis of the Ten Commandments. These commandments were not however laid down by God at this time they came about through evolution. Those men that developed these attributes would be the men that survived. We would see a system of basic rules between people. This system was not however spoken for there was no language. The system was naturally set in the human mind in the layer of behavioural programming from this time in evolution.

With the concept of personal territory came the concept of trespass. There developed unease in the mind when trespassing on another man's territory, which would serve to keep people within their own land. This unease still exists in the mind today and there is an innate guilt complex felt when trespassing on another person's property. The concept of stealing was born. By trespassing and taking food from another man's territory survival of the human race was threatened. There developed a guilt complex in the mind against stealing from another person's land.

The concept of adultery was born. This guilt complex again served the purpose of keeping people apart. Although it may have been tempting to nip over to the neighbour's wife this kind of activity did not serve to ensure survival of the human race. Firstly it could be hazardous if you got caught and it also tempted people to live closer together. With the concept of monogamy people could be confident that the sheer effort involved in raising young was directed at their own children. The people that developed this concept at this time were the ones that survived.

A further complex developed that would help ensure survival of the human race and that was against killing other human beings. Those people that did kill one and other died, which I suppose is fairly obvious. However this particular aversion to killing fellow human beings was essential in the survival of the race. There was always somebody that either had better territory or a more attractive wife. Had this aversion to killing each other not developed there would have been very few people left at this point in evolution. There weren't many of us as it was. Some estimates derived from genetic research have put the original human population at around a few thousand.

We have the idea of accepting what a man owned or had and being satisfied with it at least to the point of not killing to get something better. There was always another man again with better territory or a more attractive wife to be envied. This was controlled by a natural acceptance of one's lot and not coveting what somebody else had. This prevented conflict between people.

This was a time when there was only honesty. Dishonesty would come to be when language developed in a future time. For now there was only what was and what was not. There were no accounts spoken by people to be believed or not believed and no opportunity to lie. There was only what could be seen by a man's own eyes. The personality created in this time was totally honest. Truth was all there was.

A further change that occurred was with children. Once they grew up it was essential that they moved away or took over the parent's territory. The parents however did not die as soon as the children reached maturity. This would lead to conflict between parents and children and the teenage rebellion was born. This tormented relationship still exists today and it served a purpose in evolution and that was to spread the population out. The children would leave to find their own territories and sexual partners. There would develop an innate respect in the child for the parent. Although there would be conflict between the two the child would not challenge for the parents territory. This served the purpose of spreading the gene pool.

The natural behaviour that was set in the mind at this point in evolution for the purposes of survival formed the basis for the simple behaviour rules set out in the Ten Commandments. These rules setting aside the religious worship ones are:

Honour the Father and Mother
Not to Kill
Not to commit adultery
Not to steal
To be honest and not bear false witness against the neighbour
Not to covert the neighbours assets

These rules would form the basis of the profession of law we know today. Law was based on simple natural rules that lead to the survival of the human race. These rules still govern how people behave today and arise from evolution.

The evolution of sexual restriction

Sexual behaviour through this period in evolution was dramatically modified and this modification left lasting impressions in the mind. Reproduction was by necessity restricted. With such a limited food source it was impossible to feed a large family of children. The biology of the body hadn't significantly changed from earlier times however the mind did change. Sexual desire was restricted through stress and this restriction became etched on the mind. This process happened by natural selection. The families that didn't adapt in this way simply starved and died out. This phase of sexual restriction is recorded in the Bible.

Genesis chapter 3 reads:

7 And the eyes of them both were opened and they knew that they were naked and they sewed fig leaves together and made themselves aprons.
8 And they heard the voice of the LORD God walking in the garden in the cool of the day and Adam and his wife hid themselves from the presence of the LORD God amongst the trees of the garden.
9 And the LORD God called unto Adam, and said unto him, where art thou?
10 And he said I heard thy voice in the garden and I was afraid, because I was naked and I hid myself.
11 And he said Who told thee that thou wast naked? Hast thou eaten of the tree, whereof I commanded thee that thou shouldest not eat?
12 And the man said, the woman whom thou gavest to be with me, she gave me of the tree, and I did eat.
13 And the LORD God said unto the woman, what is that thou hast done? And the woman said The serpent beguiled me and I did eat.

14 And the LORD God said unto the serpent. Because thou hast done this, thou art cursed above all cattle and above every beast of the field; upon thy belly shalt thy go, and dust shalt thou eat all the days of thy life.

15 And I will put enmity between thee and the woman, and between thy seed and her seed; it shall bruise thy head and thou shalt bruise his heel

16 Unto the woman he said I will greatly multiply thy sorrow and thy conception; in sorrow thou shalt bring forth children; and thy desire shall be to thy husband, and he shall rule over thee.

17 And unto Adam he said thou hast hearkened unto the voice of thy wife, and hast eaten of the tree, of which I commanded thee, saying, Thou shalt not eat of it; cursed is the ground for thy sake; in sorrow shalt thou eat of it all the days of thy life.

18 Thorns also and thistles shall it bring forth to thee; and thou shalt eat the herb of the field.

The references made in the Bible have sexual connotations and refer to sexual behaviour. Fig leaves were used to cover genitals to reduce potential sexual stimulation. "Man was tempted by woman into eating the forbidden fruit". This term is commonly referred to as having sex rather than acquisition of knowledge referred to in the Bible. "Woman was tempted by the serpent", which was the penis. Enmity was expressed between the penis and woman and the concept of sex being painful written. The expression " it shall bruise thy head and thou shalt bruise his heel" refers to sex at this point in evolution. Sex was a quick affair with insufficient foreplay to arouse the female to a sufficient level of arrousement for sex not to be painful. The expression "thy desire shall be to thy husband" refers to the monogamous relationship between man and woman. The last two paragraphs quoted refer to the harsh environment, which gave rise to this concept of sexual restriction.

Sexual restriction has formed a large part of religious teaching and does provide practical benefit. It has not however been the case through all human evolution and only naturally occurred in the harshest times. This restriction has survived in the programming of the original mind. This is not to say earlier sexual behaviours are completely overwritten because they are not. There is however a natural guilt complex arising from the programming of this period that serves to help prevent sex outside monogamous relationships. The guilt complex will not always serve to prevent extra curricular activity but on the whole it will curtail it to a substantial extent when looking at a whole population. This type of sexual behaviour is not actually essential in modern living with food being in plentiful supply. It has to be remembered however that the original human mind is not actually programmed for life in the modern world. It retains its programming from the Stone Age in a period of great austerity and still behaves as though that austerity exists now - well at least some of us do.

A further natural aid to restrict procreation came with the original children that were born. These were not easy-going kids just as their parents weren't easy-going. The children were demanding because they had inherited the natural need to think for themselves. They were energetic because natural selection chose those people that kept on the go. Today small families still suit original minds more naturally than large ones. There is a requirement for substantial effort in the rearing of children and it is not an easy job. Our expectations are distorted by our sexuality, which underneath is promiscuous and comes from our time in the trees. In that period rearing children was relatively easy because of the abundant supply of fruit. This period was the opposite extreme.

Although life was extremely hard here there was one thing that wasn't essential in this place and that was complete physical fitness. There was no running anymore as the predators and other hominoids had left this place.

Furthermore the lifestyle of limited food intake and limited sexual activity contributed to the body's longevity. Today we have been long aware that a relatively meagre diet and abstinence from sex prolongs life. It may mean a long life but a rather dull one. Because of this something extraordinary occurred. This man passed the point of natural death that his body had previously been programmed for. Although the body didn't experience death the mind went through the experience. This is known today as the mid life crisis.

The mid life crisis is a natural phenomenon. The term mid life however is a little misleading. Today people commonly live into there seventies and eighties and this is where the term comes from. The crisis occurs around the age of thirty-five to forty the mid point of modern life expectancy. Looking back through even relatively recent history however average life expectancy has previously been much shorter than this. Talking from personal experience there is a significant decline in the body's fitness from around the age of 35. This is around the age most footballers get a bit long in the tooth to play at the top level. Once the body was in a state of decline in the natural world, where it was the survival of the fittest, I am afraid your days were numbered. This is where the midlife crisis comes from and is in fact naturally an end of life crisis.

Man meets God

With the mind going through the experience of death it was now that man met with God whilst still being alive. He was ordained to live on and would do so with God by his side. He did not give up and die although in all other respects he should have done so. He derived strength from his belief and confidence. There were no other men to turn to for comfort at this time and this man didn't need them for he had God. Woman on the other hand did have somebody to turn to and that was man. He dealt with future and she looked to him for guidance. Religious worship reflects this original beginning in the way people pray to God. There is a natural reason for men occupying positions as religious leaders. There is a one to one relationship with a person trying to commune with God. Man now had his soul as he had found God.

Genesis chapter 2 reads:

7. And the Lord God formed man of the dust of the ground, and breathed into his nostrils the breath of life; and man became a living soul.

This is the second creation of man in the Bible and the relevance of this second creation comes from this phase in man's evolution. This phase is distinct from the clever running man who was the first creation of man in the Bible. This man was the clever running man's descendant but this man had belief in God.

The basic religious concepts would now be formed. "God created the heaven and the earth". Man interpreted these concepts out of what he could observe and the only places he could see were the ground where he lived and the skies above him. There was an ancient mental link in the mind with the skies and death. This came from the time of the dinosaurs when the ancestor of man was carried in death to the skies by the pterosaurs. It would be this link and these places that formed the basis of religious belief in heaven and hell. Hell however was not a place to go to after death. This man already lived in hell and the concept of hell itself came from man's very existence on earth at the time of great austerity. This life however was made bearable by the very belief in going to a better place after living on earth was over. God's reward for enduring this hardship was to be given as passage to the heavens after death. This place was in the skies and he could see his ancestors had already made it to this place. They shone as stars in the night sky as they looked down upon him. The concept of heaven came to be and death was the only way to this other place and something to be welcomed when man's time for living on earth was finished.

This ability to believe is a fundamental characteristic of the original mind. This belief may true or it may not. We now know that stars are not ancestors in heaven; however at this time this was the most logical conclusion to arrive at. This belief would be the foundation for astrology, which we still use today. It is fairly clear that the movement of planets and the patterns of stars can have no influence on our lives. However think of these entities as ancestors in heaven trying to guide our lives and then astrology makes some sense. There was no influence from other men in deriving belief it was arrived at from within. This in turn also meant that convincing this mind that a belief wasn't true by external means would not be something it naturally understood and would require substantial effort.

The original man never worked with other men. Most of the modern social attributes didn't exist. There was no need for them. There was just survival. There were no people other than the family to interact with. There was no hierarchy and no status. Each man held his territory through his own skills and effort. There was a natural respect for other people. The most important survival attribute of all was obsession. Those men that had the ability to keep on going in the obsessive search for food were the men that survived. The legacy of this time would be imprinted on to all subsequent human minds with the single family forming the backbone of group living. This legacy would serve to create the characteristics that would eventually give human domination of the world. We have the creation of the autistic or original mind. The relative difference between this personality and the other human personality comes from the next phase in evolution. This is the evolution of tribal human behaviour.

Chapter Twelve

The tribe of men

Coming forward in time the world began to warm again and the rain returned. Climate studies have shown that from 130,000 years ago to 115,000 years ago the world's climate underwent a warm moist period. The rain forests expanded and deserts were almost completely covered in vegetation. This 15,000-year period would see the next great phase in our history. This was the evolution of the tribe.

The savannah began to return and food became easier to find. The larger animals returned. For there to be a start in the change from the single family existence, food must have started to be easier to find. A tribe can only be supported on an area where a reasonable quantity of game can be found. There was to come a time of plenty for all and with it an expansion in the human population. More importantly however there would be a change to group behaviour with the single-family giving way to a tribal existence. The single-family existence would however not die out completely.

Two brothers formed themselves into a binary group to find women. This was an advantage of numbers over the single-family existence. A single man could not protect his woman or daughters when faced with two men. This behaviour is reflected in the modern day. There is a distinct human discomfort in going out alone to find women. This is because hunting for females would have been a particularly dangerous activity. It's still not that safe now.

These two men however did not split up after they had found their women. As more food was available it was no longer essential for the human population to be as spread out. They stayed together with their women and this was the beginning of the tribe. Together these men cooperated as brothers and this cooperation gave them evolutionary advantage over the single-family. They were able to take and hold territory with their numerical strength. They cooperated in hunting which lead to greater success as larger and quicker animals began to reappear. They had safety in numbers and greater confidence. The previous layer of programming from the single-family began to be overwritten. These values started to fade under the new layer of behaviour that was forming.

Tribal behaviour developed through genetic selection and the groups of men grew in number that evolved this behaviour. As cooperative behaviour developed larger prey could be killed. More women could be acquired and fed. No longer was life quite as risky as it used to be and it was a little bit easier. The tribe came to be. Man's relatives had done this before and group living is a natural primate activity. Only in a time of extreme hardship was the single-family existence the most effective way of surviving. The previous programming was not lost but clouded over with the new layer of natural instructions. This new programming would be tribal human behaviour.

To be successful as a tribe of men some of the old ways had to change. No longer could man be quite so focused and obsessed. He had to think about the other men around him and what they were doing. Over time through genetic selection the natural intuition men had for knowing what their prey would do changed. This intuition became an intuition for knowing what each other would do. This developed into hierarchy with each person having their place in the order.

Most people today have the natural understanding of social order and respect hierarchy. They may not like it but they do naturally understand it. People accept what they are told by someone higher than them as being correct. They accept instructions from people in authority and do as they are told. This is not universally the case for there are a group of people that have not naturally developed this tribal concept and those people are described by the autistic or original personality.

The women developed the same intuition of what each other would do. Tribal women created a hierarchy just the same as tribal men. This hierarchy was based on sexual appeal. They competed to be the most attractive. This hierarchy is still reflected in modern life and this now takes the form of dressing to look attractive and using makeup. The female hierarchy in the tribe served the purpose of spreading the women between the men. Without hierarchy all the women would want to be with the leader of the tribe as he was the strongest male.

By necessity the tribal attributes of man were born. Only the tribes that developed these attributes survived. Unless there is some natural understanding of hierarchy a tribe just can't work. If everybody were fighting to be leader, which is the obvious position to choose, the tribe would not function. This was a time before rules so there has to be a natural understanding of position or else there would only be the best fighter left. He wouldn't be able to feed lots of women on his own.

Status was born. Somebody had to lead the tribe and there had to be a reason for him to do it. The highest status man would have first access to food and first choice in women. The strongest and fittest man took the lead. This was a time of plenty and intelligence was not critical for survival. The critical factor for survival was the ability of the tribe to work together as a single body and status was integral and essential to its functioning.

Competitiveness came to be. Status would be derived by competitiveness. The most competitive would take the lead. This would be based on fighting ability however so as not to risk serious injury it would become ritualised. This kind of behaviour is the same as in the animal kingdom where fighting between males for the right to mate does not tend to be to the death. Physical strength would be important along with size as well as speed. Wrestling would be the kind of activity that would be the way in which status in the tribe would be established.

Cruelty was born. Status could be achieved by demonstrating just how dangerous and vicious a man could be without risking death. Cruelty served the purpose of creating order through fear. At this time in evolution cruelty was quite limited because life was relatively easy and the human population was not under pressure. Cruelty would start with animals and in time this would spread to cruelty to humans. The concept of cruelty was part of the formation of the tribal mind and served an evolutionary purpose of creating order and discipline in the tribe. Cruelty in modern life is reflected in the stick part of the carrot and stick approach to motivation. It forms an integral part of maintaining discipline although it has to be carefully balanced. An excess of cruelty can prove counter productive.

The evolutionary balance to cruelty that developed was compassion for other members of the tribe. This compassion served to protect the weaker people. This was necessary in the tribe because if only the strongest were kept this would lead to a single person and the tribe could not function. In the modern world compassion is extended well beyond compassion for fellow tribal members however this is cultural rather than natural. The natural compassion humans have is limited to a tribal scale.

Pride came to be. A man could feel proud if he was successful in the eyes of other men. Pride was necessary in the tribe to get men to work hard enough for survival. This pride would take the form of pride in actions and status within the tribe. As far as actions are concerned pride would come from successful contribution to the hunting effort. Being the man that made the kill would derive the greatest pride of all. This behaviour is reflected in football. The man that gets the goal derives the greatest adulation. However because team effort was what mattered in the tribe the pride was spread through each man's contribution to the hunt. The man that found the prey would receive adulation, as would those that blocked the prey's escape. This adulation would be less than for the man who made the kill; however these men would derive the feeling of pride when they made a successful contribution to the hunt. The whole tribe was motivated into successful team effort by the concept of pride.

There was also the concept of pride in a man's status within the tribe. This form of pride was a longer-term motivator. Sustained success in the hunt could lead to a man gaining elevation in status. He would feel proud of his elevation and this would motivate further effort towards the success of the tribe. In today's society pride is obtained from successful effort in the same way. It is the carrot part of the carrot and stick approach, reflected in rewards and awards. Pride from status is derived from career progression provided that progression is upwards and not downwards.

Self-awareness evolved along with pride and status. People became aware of who they were within the group. They now had a position and an image to consider in front of other people and in order to maintain these things they had to become aware of themselves. This self-awareness precluded actions and words that didn't fit with what other people found comfortable and embarrassment evolved to curtail excess. This would serve to provide a unifying level of behaviour that ensured the tribe functioned as one.

Loyalty was another human attribute that developed to cement people together. Those tribes with loyal members developed better social cohesion and stood a better chance of success. This loyalty would be to the leader and to the tribe in general. These people naturally despised disloyalty and any member that was seen to be disloyal would have to endure the hatred expressed by the other tribal members. The human characteristic of loyalty to their tribe formed an important function in evolution and was naturally written down in the tribal mind.

Sexual prowess came to be. The tribe would have sex in front of each other. The better a man was seen at satisfying women the more women he could potentially have sex with. Sexual prowess would serve to create balance and restrict aggression from taking rule. If the tribe were purely based on aggression only the best fighter would have sex. This form of behaviour can be seen in animals. Man isn't physically adapted to live like this. Hence Sexual prowess is an important element in tribal living. Penis size is important to display to the female the pleasure available. The ability not to ejaculate too quickly is important so that the female achieves satisfaction from intercourse and wants more.

A new form of love between adults was born. These personal attachments protected the genes of individuals and made sure that not just the leader had children. Love serves to protect individual's genes. Tribal love developed to be more intense than the earlier form. Passion was increased with a greater demonstration of this love. This served the purpose of display to the tribe so that other members understood that these people were in love and not to interfere in this relationship. This demonstration took the form of kissing, being close together, holding hands and caressing each other. They would sleep close together at night so that each could be sure that the other was being faithful.

The tribal form of love with its increased level of passion would make the earlier form of love from the single-family existence look distinctly icy and cold in comparison. The increased level of passion and the associated pleasure that went with love did mean that love in the tribe became a more sought after experience. This would lead to a number of relationships rather than the one as in the earlier single-family existence. Tribal love was more intense; however that intensity lasted for a shorter time.

Love served the purpose of creating reason for everybody to be in the tribe.

With group cooperation came the need for a tool to coordinate the tribe. There was a need for each man to know what other men were doing in the hunt and what he should do. As groups of men grew in number intuition and ancient gesticulation was no longer sufficient to coordinate activity. The tool that came to be was language. Language is sophisticated and as such I believe was a late development in human evolution. Prior to this point change had been very slow with simple tools based on observation gradually changing over hundreds of thousands of years. Language on the other hand is an abstract concept. Even today it is difficult and time consuming to learn. I believe that language evolved in the tribe and the natural understanding of it forms part of the tribal mind.

With the development of language came some of the more advanced abstract human concepts. One of these concepts is dishonesty. A lie could only exist between two people and it needed language to communicate it. Prior to this point people only understood what they could see with their own eyes. There was only the natural concept of honesty in the single-family. Now with language there was the opportunity to obtain information indirectly from another person. This information could however be relayed in altered form if that alteration served advantage to the person relaying it. The lie was born. Lying served a useful purpose in preventing upset and discontent and those tribes that learned to lie to a certain extent found they had better social cohesion. The ability to lie though had its natural boundaries and taken to excess would be counter productive. These boundaries were what we term "white lies" today. These are little untruths, which prove beneficial in human relationships and not detrimental.

Along with language came humour in the form of jokes. Humour served to diffuse potential conflicts between

94

people and create social cohesion. In the tribe not everybody will have the same point of view, as there is a hierarchy. Humour serves the purpose of getting a message across without causing offence. We use humour today in just the same way. There is generally a message in a joke.

Sociability and recreation developed along with an increase in pleasure in being in others company. People could work a little less hard because the tribal existence was more successful than the previous existence. With large kills there was spare time as there was no point in killing something else because it would only go rotten before it could be eaten. These pleasures were expressed in a number of forms. There was pleasure in story telling. The adventures of the hunters would be recanted to the other tribal members probably at some length and perhaps with a fair degree of tedium however it was a good idea to look interested. The children would love the stories and look up to the hunters and wish they could be like these heroes some day. There was pleasure in gossip and banter. The opportunity now arose to discuss what other people were doing and pleasure taken from generally disapproving of others actions. There was pleasure in dance. This would serve as sexual display but also as a tool to bind the tribe together so they acted as one. Each member would dance to the same rhythm and be able to keep to that rhythm. There was pleasure in displaying ones status when eating. The highest status would eat first followed by the next highest and so on down through the tribe.

With language and story telling people started to learn from other people's words. This is the start of tribal learning, which is distinctly different from the previous form of learning purely by observation. The man with the highest status would be the person to copy in order to try and achieve his level of success. People would listen to what he had to tell them and try to use this information to improve their own success. This form of learning

95

dominated for a very long time. In the future the spoken word would be translated into the written word, which would form vast libraries of knowledge. Today many books are sold are on the basis of the status of the author. These books include ones by celebrities and politicians. It is the status that sells not the content of the book. People still look to high status people and want to hear what they have to say in case they themselves can learn anything from that successful person's words. It has to be said that these books can on occasion not be quite as full of gems of wisdom as might be hoped for.

The tribal form of learning was prone to a weakness and that was human distortion of reality. In the tribe the stories of the hunt would become slightly exaggerated. Instead of the tribe happening on an unfortunate encounter with a single decrepit old lion looking for somewhere to die in peace this event would become an encounter with a pride of savage foaming sabre toothed lions hell bent on death and destruction of man kind. The exaggeration created entertainment and it was not really in anybody's interest to undermine it. The boast was born and was an accepted part of tribal living.

It is the natural understanding of story telling that provides one of the characteristics that separates the tribal mind from the original mind. A characteristic observed in the autistic personality is a perceived lack of imagination and conceptualisation. What is really being observed is the lack of ability to turn a verbal story into images in the mind. The original mind did not evolve to learn based on stories and doesn't have a natural interest in them.

Group living in the tribe necessitated a better understanding of the feelings of others and empathy developed. This is a natural ability to see situations from another person's perspective. Empathy facilitates compromise between people - a necessary requirement for group living. With people living in close proximity to each other there developed an awareness of personal space.

There was a natural distance that people liked to have from each other to feel comfortable. There was the need for pleasantries and manners. These human characteristics helped prevent upset in the tribe and created social cohesion. Manners serve to prevent offence and pleasantries help to create comfort in the presence of other people.

This wider view of the feelings of other people meant that the previous human characteristics from the single family were overwritten with the new tribal social characteristics. The focus and obsession became clouded under this new programming. The acute senses became less acute as the other attributes became more important to survive as a tribe. No longer did vision need to take in as much information. There were many eyes to see things. The ability to bear pain increased. Fighting in the form of wrestling encouraged higher pain thresholds in successful men. In the hunt social cooperation encouraged more risks to be taken with the chance for injury increasing. No longer did injury mean certain death, as the tribe would look after those that were hurt. Hearing became less sensitive as the ability to listen to conversation became more important. The mind developed to cut out more of the background noise from other conversations in order that the relevant words could be heard. The sense of smell reduced in close living with less sensitivity to body odours of one form and another. These people didn't take baths, sweated quite a lot and didn't have toilet paper. The tribe was now a body of people functioning together as one for the common good. The human senses reduced because either they weren't needed or they were counter-productive to that common good.

The tribes of men grew in number as they developed hunting techniques. The environment would become again the domain of huge herds of herbivores grazing on the plains of grass. The tribes needed large kills to feed themselves and needed to hunt similar sized animals to the modern day cow. They hunted the huge herds of bison.

Success in killing large game required improved hunting tools. Attempting to kill a cow sized animal with a hand axe had its risks shall we say. Although this was the way relative hominoid ancestors had perhaps done it in the past it was still pretty dangerous. Man was lighter bodied than these hominoids and particularly vulnerable to his bones being broken. To compensate a tool was developed that was in effect an elongated canine tooth. This tool was the spear and it propelled the tribes to success. This was not a new innovation because relative hominoids also had spears. It was however all but essential for big game hunting and man now needed this tool. With plenty of food derived from successful hunting techniques the tribes would come to dominate the plains. Earliest known finds of Homo Sapiens date from around 120,000 years ago which is the time I believe the tribes had expanded the human population to a significant level.

Chapter Thirteen

The time of hardship and the union of the tribe and the family

The original man and his single-family existence didn't die out despite the tribe's dominance of the plains. He continued to survive in his single-family group as he had done before. In chapter sixteen we will look in more detail at autistic characteristics of the descendents of the original family to show that this mind exists today.

As the tribe evolved socially and took in effect a socialist route the single-family evolved and took a capitalist route. The original mind hadn't fundamentally changed from that set in the time of great austerity in the desert. Food was now easier to find and this would lead to a slow change in lifestyle that would lead the single-family from being hunters to farmers. The original single-family was shy and kept out of the way of the tribe. A barrier would develop in behavioural differences that would serve to keep that separation in place. The tribe had social skills and the single family didn't. The single-family seemed like crude unpleasant people that were not nice. The tribe and the single family had very little in common other than they looked the same. They had very little to do with each other. Each had there own type of animal they hunted. The tribe hunted big game and the single-family small game.

The original man's basic make up remained the same, obsessive, focussed with acute senses. He still retained his natural sense with his prey. Whilst the tribe developed its hunting skills with spears he still killed in the same way he had always done with a hand axe to the throat. There was no need to change for he did not hunt big game. The tribe would develop better coordination with their use of spears. They would become better throwers and more acurate. They would develop a better sense of distance judgement. In a future time this would lead to a better natural ability to throw and catch balls in their descendents.

The original family developed their relationship with their prey. Home was in foothills of the mountains where there was vegetatation in the form of coarse grasses. On this vegatation lived an animal that was the ancestor of the modern day goat. The original family would adapt and this creature would eventually become their main source of food. The single-family's natural understanding of what this prey would do developed into a close relationship with this creature. There was compassion for the animal and an understanding of its needs. The original family developed this close relationship to the point of living with these creatures. They were now part of the original family and these people were now farmers.

The single-family was wealthy in food. They were never hungry now. They had much more than they needed and they were the first capitalists. Their animals were now their property and seen as such. The original family would try and defend their animals and scare predators away. When animals were killed for food this was perfomed in the most humane way possible so as to cause as little distress to the animal and the flock. It is distress caused in killing that leads to the fear of predators by their prey. The original family overcame this distress and fear by keeping the animal calm as the throat was cut. This form of killing became very refined and quick. This form of slaughter would in time become so respected it would find its way into religion. The tool used in slaughter that being the hand axe would come to be respected in a way that the spear was not. In a future time the hand axe would become the sword. This weapon would be associated with honour.

The time of plenty would however only last for the original-family with its capitalist lifestyle. The tribe on the other hand would come to a time of hardship. This hardship arose out of a change in the environment to more arid conditions along with an expansion in the tribal population. What happened next in the human evolutionary story would become so important it would find its way into religion. The original human personality would now gain status in the eyes of the tribal human personality. Rather than being reviled as happened in the time of plenty it would come to be worshiped in the time of hardship.

From around 110,000-90,000 years ago the world was undergoing a cooling period with conditions becoming more arid. Part of this phase was very arid and I believe it was this time that saw the union of the tribe and the family. Today both personalities exist together and we need to find reason for that.

The tribe had become specialists in hunting big game in the form of bison. These animals however came under severe pressure from the environment. The lush grass plains they roamed were becoming dry and arid. The bison were falling in number dramatically and the tribes were losing their staple food source. There was also a human attribute that was now lost to the tribe. This attribute was innovation.

The tribes had eventualy evolved to be not very innovative. The very existence of status precluded innovation. It was bad for a man in the tribes to be seen doing something the tribe didn't think he should be doing. These men had to think of their status. Mistakes could mean loosing position in the eyes of other men. It was bad to be seen making mistakes. Men had to fit in. To do this they had to do the same as other people in the tribe. These men didn't now have the genetic make up to innovate sufficiently in these times of hardship. The tribal mind now learned from what people had said before even if what had been said was wrong or didn't suit a new situation. The tribes were hungry and needed food. It would be now that some tribes became more aggressive in the competition for food, some would leave and some would turn to God in their time of need.

Homo sapien remains have been found at Qafzeh in the Middle East dating from 100,000 years ago and further remains found at mount Carmel in Israel dated at 80,000 years old. These were the first Homo sapien migrants and they left Africa in search of food. This time frame coincides with a period of global cooling. This change in behaviour was driven by need rather than desire. The tribes that remained in Africa were the most competetive and held the original central territory. The first migrants to leave were the least competitive. These people would eventually find themselves pushed out to the edge of the world.

The natural understanding of what prey would do was lost to the tribe. Their natural understanding had become programmed to understand one another. There was however a man, and that is the original man, who did have this natural understanding still. He seemed to the tribe to have more energy than they did. They had become slightly less active than he as they had become more successful. The tribe started to admire the original man for his special powers with animals. The animals actually lived with him and his family, which seemed extraordinary to the tribe. He didn't have to run after them.

In the past hunting was an integral part of tribal life and enjoyable. Now hunting was marked with increasing disappointment and failure and no longer was it the pleasurable experience it once had been. Hunger acted to further depress the tribe and they fell into a spiral of misery. They increasingly looked at the original family with admiration but also fear. This family had magical powers and perhaps the tribe even thought that God looked over them and gave them his protection. The tribe could have tried to steal from the original family; however they were afraid of the power that seemed to protect them. The tribe did not steal.

The time of greatest hardship came and the tribe now approached the original family for help. They were desperately hungry and the chief was under severe pressure to do something. The tribe offered the original family their finest spears and stone tools they had made in exchange for food. The original man however had no use for these things and the tribe's offer was rejected. I believe human behaviour would have been the same then as it is today. An offer is made and would either be accepted or not. The original mind is not a natural negotiator as there was no one to negotiate with in the original single-family existence.

The tribe were however natural negotiators. They had to negotiate with each other and hence naturally did not take up a rigid unmoving position. The tribe did not give up and it increased its offer to the maximum they could give in the form of their most valuable asset. They offered something that the original man could not in the end resist. The offer was the prettiest young woman that the tribe possessed. She was beautiful absolutely perfect in every way and desired by every man in the tribe. She was a virgin and hence so valuable for the simple reason no man had had her and every man wanted her. The action of this offering would serve to underpin religious worship in a future time.

The making of offerings to God came from the original negotiations between the tribe and the original family. The concept of offerings would over time change from what originally was a commercial negotiation to a religious ritual as time served to blur reality. This blurring came about as stories passed from one generation to the next. Each time a story was passed on it became a little more exaggerated and further from the original truth. In a future time understanding would become so distorted that people would believe humans should be sacrificed as an offering to God. By this time they had a few more Gods as well, such was the distortion of truth. The concept of the offering was to give a thing of great value to God in exchange for his help. This concept all arose out of the tribe offering its most valuable thing to the original family in exchange for food.

103

The virgin girl would have significance for the future of religion. She was the tribe's icon and vehicle of communication with God. For the original family she did not have the same iconic status. She was seen as the corrupter of original values. This difference in perspective between tribal and original minds would in a future time be part of a split in the Christian church. Tribal values would look towards the virgin girl, as she was their saviour. This girl would become the Virgin Mary. The original minds would not view the virgin girl in the same light or with the same importance. These minds in the form of the protestant faith would only have Christ and God himself to look towards. The virgin girl was not their saviour. The original mind had taken her in payment for feeding the tribe. This association had taken the original family from an Eden like existence where they had more food than they could ever eat into an existence that would shape the future world. The association between the original mind and the tribal mind would often be tormented and this is reflected in the Bible in the disdain that is shown for the caving in to sexual desire. It was sexual desire that created the union between the original family and the tribe in the first place.

The original man was tormented by desire for the young woman. She was displayed before him in all her nudity. His most recent behavioural programming was to have just one woman, which came from the time of great austerity in the desert. This programming arose out of affordability however now the original man was wealthy. He also had older layers of programming from previous evolution going right back to the time of promiscuity when the ancestors lived in the trees. These different layers of behavioural programming conflicted with each other. In the end however he could not resist the allure of this woman. She was too much for any man to resist. The original man took the offer. He was however racked with guilt for what he had done. This guilt was programmed into him by natural selection for it was the monogamous men that had survived the time in the desert in the single-family existence from where all people were descended.

The first true profession was born and this was prostitution. The very concept of profession describes somebody who is paid for work done. For a profession to exist there has to be someone able to pay for it. This someone was a farmer and he was the first man of wealth in evolution. The profession would not however be seen in a very positive light even though it had saved the tribe. The original man could not seem to accept his own guilt at not being able to resist temptation. The tribe would come to resent the dependence it would have on the original family. In the middle was the girl who made the deal happen although this was through no choice of her own. She had saved her people yet she was to become resented by everybody. The first profession would always be looked down upon but it was this profession that created cooperation between the original family and the tribe. This cooperation would form the basis of the modern human world.

With the concept of trade came the need to keep accounts. We now had cause for the evolutionary selection for mathematical ability. Accountancy was born. The original family would now supply the tribe with food and this necessitated a need to keep track of livestock levels. By supplying too much food stock levels could fall dangerously low. Each animal would be counted and a mental track kept of how many animals there were in the flock. Only those families that could count would survive. This natural ability with mathematics has been passed on to the descendants of this family.

The union between the tribe and the original family was mutually beneficial although the original man's wife wasn't altogether impressed. Luckily for him she could not speak or he would have been in for a certain amount of verbal abuse. She would however make him suffer in other ways. There were the cutting hard stares, spitting in his food and a general sense of loathing that was brought to bear. His close intuition with his wife meant he felt what she felt and he suffered her pain. He knew really what he had done was wrong and he would have to suffer for it but he would not give up trying to find excuses.

In these hard and violent times the tribe could protect the original family from other tribes that were also hungry. Some of these tribes did not have reverence for the original families. They would steal and in some cases kill them. This behaviour would be self-defeating as it was unsustainable. If the flock were not managed the food would run out. These tribes would then have to move on to the next victim or die. When the victims ran out the tribe would die. The tribe that chose to trade with and protect the original family would not die. They would become soldiers and in return the original family was their farmer. The original family could afford to kill a number of animals in the flock and provide sufficient food to feed the tribe in its time of need. Together the tribe and the original family survived each relying on the other.

The relationship between the original family and the tribe would become deeply etched in to future religion. The Christ is recognised for feeding the five thousand in the New Testament. There is however no magic behind this concept. The concept simply comes from evolution and is derived from farming. It is the farmer that has the ability to feed many people. The Christ was a shepherd in the New Testament and the significance of this is that the original family were shepherds. It was a shepherd that fed the tribe in its time of need. The tribe on the other hand were suppliers of certain pleasure commodities along with protection. The tribe were soldiers and like any work a man is paid for the service he offers. Soldiers are paid today in the same way and that is to protect us. The same would have been true in the past. The original man was the first farmer and he paid for his protection with food. Farmers today still enjoy a privileged position and are paid homage in the form of subsidies. This all stems from the original beginning. The original family fed the tribe in its time of need.

The tribes with an original family had a competitive edge to survive and it was this cooperation that did ensure survival. The original family would now come into contact with the tribe on a more regular basis. The original family still lived separate as it tended its flocks but not so far away as the tribe could not defend the family when the need arose. The increased contact meant that the original family was exposed to a tool the tribe used but one the family had never needed. This tool was language. The original family would learn the tribes language but not have the natural ability with it that they had. In the tribe people had names so that a person could be identified when being spoken to and they had develped a natural ability at remembering names. The tribe also had developed a natural ability at remembering the faces that went with the names. In the original family there were no names or any need for them. There was the father the mother and the children. Neither was there a natural ability at remembering numerous different faces in the original family. There were no faces to remember in the family.

The original family didn't have the genetic make up to really understand the tribe and the tribe didn't really understand the original family. The original mind doesn't naturally have the more complex characteristics of the tribal mind and likewise the tribal mind has an altered version of the natural characteristics of the original mind. The original family were odd and quite frightening. They had no social niceties or manners. The family was not likeable because it was different. When the tribe and the family did meet the children would play together. The games were from a past time and all children had inherited the same deep-rooted interest in these games. This interest is so deep-rooted that it is just the same today and the games are the same. These games were tag and hide and seek which had evolved in the time when relative hominoid gangs hunted man. Now however children in the tribe had inherited the concept of social order. They would through their childhood practice the tools they would use in their adult life.

The tools children practiced would be learning the ability of forming alliances and small gangs. Tribal children had a natural desire to do these things for it was these abilities that ensured the functioning of the tribe. A social order would be developed amongst the children based on strength. The strongest would lead and each child would learn his and her place in the tribal order. The children of the original family did not fit in with this, as they had not inherited the natural abilities that went to create order in the tribe. The original children had no concept of what position they should occupy and neither did the tribal children know.

Some of the original children would begin to create their own unique positions within the tribe. These children formed a niche for themselves and became entertainers. The children of the tribe did not like being laughed at because they understood the concept of ridicule. Ridicule served the purpose of chastising mistakes in the tribe. The original children however had no understanding of ridicule and some of these children would become the very first comedians. They would clown around and make the children of the tribe laugh. They would create their own unique place in the hierarchy. They would be different and not really understood but they would be valued in time for their unique abilities.

A gradual integration took place between the tribal and original children. The original children lacked natural social skills but they had an attribute that the tribal children did not have. This attribute was obsession. They still had the mental make up from the time of great austerity in the desert when obsession was the key to survival. It would be obsession that would drive the tribe forwards and it would be the original children that would provide it. In the past these children would have left their parents at puberty to find their own partners and start their own single-family existence. There was however now a change and although some chose the traditional farming route some chose to become a permanent part of the tribe when they grew up. This would have an everlasting impact for the future of mankind.

The original children learnt from the tribal children tribal characteristics. These characteristics had natural innate limits in the tribal mind. The original children however had no such boundaries because the characteristics were purely learnt. This would in time lead to a stretching of the limits of behaviour. Some original children would learn to be cruel. The limits on cruelty set in the tribal mind however would not apply to these children. These children could learn to be very cruel indeed. Some children would take an interest in tool making. They however were not limited by tribal ways. They would not be afraid of making mistakes or being laughed at. These children would be the ones to drive forward innovation and that innovation would be born out of obsession. This would in time lead to previously unseen technical advancement. There would also be some children that would grow old in the tribe. They would pass the point of natural physical death that the body was programmed for through evolution. These people would like their ancestors now walk with God by their side. The difference now was that they were able to communicate the experience to other people as they had leant language. These people would become religious teachers to the tribe and in time would become very influential in the evolution of the human world.

We now have the basic natural behavioural programming of people. We are not distinguished by colour or how we look. We are only different in how we think. In chapter eighteen we will carry on with the evolutionary story to gain insight into the geography of the world. For the time being however we will concentrate on the psychological characteristics of the two minds along with a look at the history surrounding research into the original mind.

Part Two

What our Evolution means to us Today.

Chapter Fourteen

Conflicting evolutionary programming and the existence of two minds

What does our evolutionary experience mean to us now? The answer is rather a lot and it in fact explains much of current human behaviour. We have been mentally programmed to survive through evolution and this programming forms what we are now. Should we be a confused species? I would say we should. Our sexual programming for instance is not singular. We have conflicting programs from different periods in evolution. We are programmed to be promiscuous from our time in the trees. On top of this however we are programmed to be monogamous from our time of great austerity in the desert.

Our diet has changed through evolution. Our first recognisable food looking at the clues from our teeth were small insects and creatures that were easily caught. We changed into fruit eaters once we took to the trees. When we became hominoids living on the ground we evolved to be carnivores living on meat. We were first active in the day as amphibian type creatures. With our mammalian form we evolved to become nocturnal. From night creatures we turned back to living in the day once we took to the trees. We have lived under the ground, over the ground and on the ground. Our evolutionary experiences have adapted us to live virtually anywhere and at any time be it day or night.

The single most important feature to come out of our evolution however is the existence of two separate types of human mind. These are the original human mind and the tribal human mind. It is the combination of the two that gives us the world we know. Without the original mind we would still be hunters living in the Stone Age as we would have had little innovation. Without the tribal mind we would also still be living in the Stone Age. We would have no concept of the naturally occurring human characteristics that allow us to function together as a group.

By understanding our evolution we can understand many of the conflicts that affect our mind. We have for an eternity as a species been in search of contentment and fulfilment. The concept that this fulfilment lies in death has some truth in it in so far as the mind ceases to function. However when you're dead you're dead and stand little chance of achieving anything. In life can fulfilment ever be truly achieved? I suspect not when you consider our evolutionary make up. One part of our evolutionary mind will always be in conflict with another part. We are programmed to have one woman and many women and likewise for the women one man and many men. We are programmed to eat lots of food from our time in the trees and very little food from our time in the desert. This gives us guilt complexes about the amount we eat. We are programmed to eat only fruit and only meat. We have a complex about what we eat. We assume that we are naturally sociable creatures and this is how we as a society should behave. In our evolution however at one of our most formative periods we were not naturally sociable creatures at all. The very existence of the single human family comes from an unsociable existence.

The existence of two basic human minds today

Now there is a question that I have not yet touched on and that is a combination of the two mind types in one person. There have been countless opportunities for the crossing of the two since they were formed in Africa. The question is would such a crossing result in one or the other being produced as in say, somebody with blue eyes having sex with somebody with brown eyes and the resultant baby having blue or brown eyes rather than a mix of the two colours. Or would the crossing result in a mix of mental characteristics as in a black person having sex with a white person producing a brown baby. My inclination would be towards a mix of mental characteristics being formed by a cross of the original and tribal mind. When we think of society, as a whole, there isn't an obvious discrete split but rather a continuum and range to human personality. Different people to different degrees display different characteristics from the two basic personalities. There are however still two identifiably separate mind types towards the ends of a whole spectrum of human personality. This leads me to believe that both have survived without crossing. There are factors within the two basic personalities that have served to prevent this happening.

The factors that have helped keep the two mind types apart are a natural connection between original minds and a separate natural connection between tribal minds. The two do not tend to be drawn to each other. The tribal mind will tend to be more concerned with attractiveness. The original mind won't tend to be as bothered about attractiveness. This arises from there being more sexual competition in the tribe than in the single-family existence and the existence of choice.

The original mind in women will be looking for a special connection and commitment that they will tend to find in an original man. They are naturally programmed for a monogamous relationship that is life long. Temptation is restricted by a more profound sense of guilt in cheating. For the tribe it was different. Sexual relationships were not monogamous for life and the very concept of sexual prowess comes from there being choice.

To the original mind the tribal mind can seem boring. To the tribal mind the original mind can seem geeky and odd. Location also serves to separate the two. On a world scale there are different balances of concentrations in different countries. Religion has played its part in keeping the mind types separate. Certain religions appeal more to original minds and others more to tribal minds. For instance the Jewish religion and Puritanical Christian faith such as Quakerism tend to have more appeal to the natural values of the original mind. The Muslim religion and Catholic faith are better suited to the tribal mind.

The character of the two minds

The natural character of the two basic mind types are distinctly different however this is not as easy to observe as it might be. The reason for this is partly due to the crossing of the two but is also due to learnt behaviour.

The natural character of the original mind should still reflect the attributes necessary for survival in the original way of life. The original single-family existence in the desert programmed the original mind for a hard life. Not only was that life hard it was also monotonous with most of the time spent in the search of food. Obsession was the key to survival. It was those families that obsessively searched for food that survived. This means the characteristics should be much simpler than for the tribal mind although you might not think this when you meet one.

The natural social characteristics are missing in the original mind which means interaction can seem a bit odd. I have experienced for instance the single sentence that lasts about an hour with apparently no breathing involved. On the other hand there can be virtually no communication and extracting even the shortest of sentences can be a painful experience. There is a lack of natural understanding of how conversation works with each person taking their turn. This can lead to very one sided interactions with an apparent lack of listening involved.

The original mind should be particularly active because the activity level necessary for survival in the original single-family existence was high. The senses should be heightened because it was only in the tribe that they were

115

toned down. These senses also vary according to temporary mental activity levels. The higher the level of mental activity the more sensitive the body becomes. The mind will tend to be more aware of noise, touch, vision and smell. There may be varying balances of these senses from one person to the next. Some people may be more aware of noise for instance or comfort than others. I haven't managed quite yet to fully work out the logic behind the different balance of the senses from one person to the next - maybe some day.

The original mind should demonstrate a high level of focus although this should only be typically reflected in the male mind. This focus is derived from following the tracks of animals in the desert. The female mind had a different purpose in the original existence, which was much wider ranging. She looked after children and searched for food at the same time. This is commonly called multi tasking which women have inherited the ability to do. This mind will naturally be honest as there was nobody to deceive or lie to in the original existence. It will seem to be less compliant because natural compromise evolved in the tribe. This mind above all shouldn't stop thinking and demonstrate some degree of obsession, the reason above all that ensured survival of the human species.

The natural character of the tribal mind will feature the more complex attributes necessary for a tribal existence. These features will include an awareness of social status on a tribal scale. This means there is a natural understanding of position within a group. There should exist a natural understanding of the other necessary features of tribal living. These include on the positive side tribal love, compassion, loyalty, and kindness. On the negative side there's cruelty, vindictiveness, dishonesty and jealousy.

Personal attractiveness is an important feature in the tribal mind. In the tribe there was competition for sex and choice. The most attractive men and women were the ones that attracted higher demand for sex. Choice meant that sexual relations weren't limited to a single partner for life but multiple partners. There should be a natural awareness of recreation in the tribal mind. Life in the tribe was relatively easy and it wasn't a case of all work and no play. Play or recreation served to pass the time when there was no need to hunt. Pride should be a feature in this mind. Pride in one's position and ability was important to make the tribe function together with each member performing their duties to the best of their abilities. There is competitiveness and pleasure from winning. People competed against each other for improved social status. Tribes competed with each other for territory. Competition drove evolution and it drove the evolution of the tribe.

Language is a feature where there should be a difference between the two minds. This is however difficult to see clearly as only fairly basic language is likely to have existed at the end of substantive natural selection. The rest of ability with language is learnt. Even in recent times language has evolved substantially. English from five hundred years ago is significantly different to English now.

There should however according to our evolutionary story be a wider range of ability in the original mind because there is no innate bottom line to fall back on and obsession with language at the other extreme. Language in this mind will range from simple to complex. I remember an old farmer who used to visit our house for Sunday dinner when I was little. It was very rare for him to string two words together. It would be" yup" and "nope" and that's about all you ever got out of him. This was in his genetic make up. He had an original mind and had never really learnt to talk much. He worked on his own and lived with his brother and sister. He had only ever lived a family existence like the original man. At the other extreme I look at Thomas Hardy. Have you ever read one of his books? In his case it is genius although I couldn't get past the first page his descriptions were so elaborate. In the hands of lesser men the over use of language turns into waffle.

There's plenty of that around today. Waffle should be more likely in the original mind although it can be copied by the tribal mind in the mistaken belief that waffle is a sign of intellect. Waffle is just waffle I'm afraid and I hope I haven't done too much of it.

There should remain the natural understanding and closeness to animals for the original mind. This closeness comes from the intimate relationship that the original family had with the natural world and further evolved to have with their livestock. This close relationship manifests itself in different ways in modern society. Pets are likely to be a feature and there should be an aversion to animal cruelty. In farmers with original minds there will be a close connection with livestock and its welfare. In children with original minds there should be an interest in animals and a level of compassion for welfare that shouldn't be seen naturally in the tribal mind.

As far as the more complex natural tribal characteristics are concerned they can all be learnt by the original mind. Like language this should lead to a wide range with virtually no appreciation at the bottom end and an extreme understanding at the top end when combined with obsession. If competitiveness is learnt and combined with obsession this can lead to exceptional performance. Likewise with any of the characteristics of the tribal mind the original mind can perform over a full range. The original mind can be very loving or it can appear to show no love at all. Likewise with the negative emotions the original mind could have no vindictiveness at all and at the other extreme be very vindictive indeed. It can show no cruelty at all or at the other extreme in the wrong environment be extremely cruel indeed. From a visit I made to Romania it appeared to me that Vlad the Impaler had a particularly bad upbringing. He developed a very nasty habit of sticking people on spikes.

One of the fundamental differences between the two minds is the process by which decisions are taken. The

118

original mind perceives two choices and sees either black or white. This comes from the original existence where this mind was the maker of all decisions. There were no other people to consider or contribute to the decision making process. The original man either did something or he didn't and that was it. The tribal mind in addition to black and white also sees a shade of grey or doubt. This originates from the tribal existence. Other people had to be considered and be allowed to contribute to the decision making process. This creates the area of grey in this mind due to the fact that the opinions of other people are unknown. The tribal mind has this natural doubt and needs the contribution of others to arrive at certainty.

Understanding of human behavior has up until now been based on the concept of there being a single personality with variation from a perceived normal behavior attributed to mental dysfunction. As far as high functioning autism, in the form of "Asperger's Syndrome", is concerned this variation is thought of as a developmental disorder. However that understanding is not correct and is based on fundamentally flawed principles. In the case of lower functioning autism I consider that a developmental disorder could be considered true but only to the extent that learning ability is disrupted. The prospect of autism being due to a brain abnormality through genetic fault, brain insult or brain disease is in my view extremely unlikely. The basic personality is normal and is only considered abnormal through the mistaken and amoral concept of eugenics, which we will look at next.

Chapter Fifteen

Scientific observation of the original mind

The classification of Asperger's Syndrome as a mental disorder is fundamentally flawed because it is based on political rather than real science. In such circumstances it is only possible to accept such work in the field of human behaviour if we accept the political motivations that went with it. Society draws the line between normal and abnormal based on its values of the time with psychology and philosophy merging as one. Asperger's Syndrome rather than being a mental disorder in fact constitutes a political disorder based on the misconceived concept of eugenics.

Hans Asperger carried out his initial observations of the original mind during the Second World War in Nazi Austria. The resulting thesis entitled "Die "Autitischen Psychopathen" im Kindesalter" (Autistic Psychopathy in Childhood) was entered for publication on the 8th October 1943. Hans Asperger was the director of "Heilpadagogischen Abteilung der Klinic" (The Clinic's Department of Orthopaedaogogy) at the University of Vienna under the presidency of a one Professor Franz Hamburger.

To see the Nazi doctrine that motivated the work we need to look to the man that Asperger worked under. This was Franz Hamburger. The following account reproduced in its entirety comes from a leading Medical Journal of the time. Its correspondent to Berlin wrote the article on March 27th 1939 and it was published shortly afterwards under the foreign letters section. We can see a clear picture of the reality of the situation that Asperger was working in.

"The New Wiener Medizinische Gesellschaft"

"In the train of events under the new regime in Austria the famous Gesellschaft der Aerzte, like many other time-honoured organisations, has lately been dissolved. In 1937 the centenary of the society was celebrated in a manner befitting so illustrious a medical body. The greatest German names in the world of medicine enthusiastically participated in this celebration. The list of speakers and scientific lecturers was brilliant and in keeping with the accomplishments of the society and its reputation. But its continuance was not to be tolerated by the Nazi rulers of Vienna, and, like all the other medical societies, it was disestablished, in the 101st year of its existence. In its stead a new Wiener medizinsche Gesellschaft was created, designed to serve medical practitioners and scientific research. Naturally only Aryan doctors are admitted to membership and in addition foreigners who are unquestionably in sympathy with the regime. The plan of the new society includes sections for the various special disciplines to take the place of the former societies of specialists. There is also newly added a special section for military medicine. The president of the new society is no distinguished clinician; he is the Nazi district governor of Vienna, that is to say a politician who is also an official of the Nazi bureau of national health.

In his inaugural address, February 4, the new president himself stated that he was well aware that many representatives of science were not wholly in accord with the establishment of the new organisation under political rather than under scientific auspices. The president is Dr O. Planner-Plan. This political control has become necessary, he stated, because as district governor he is better informed about local public health affairs than anyone else. Since he has the representatives of science at his beck and call, it is possible for him to draw on consultant opinion in any problem which may arise. As he put it, "Prominent representatives of the various specialities may be commissioned to give an opinion with regard to any questions, and thus their abundant knowledge will be made to serve the nations health." Dr.

Planner-Plan's address was embroidered with a wealth of detail, which may be briefly summarized: The present speedy tempo of the national work program in Germany not only should be maintained but should be surpassed. This means that a maximal expenditure of energy will be demanded of all German workers and soldiers. A further objective is conservation of the prolonged efficiency of the nations workers. In this connection the physicians have an important mission to fulfil. Specialising physicians, too, have their respective duties, which the president went on to enumerate.

At each session of the new society a lecture and demonstrations will be given. It is further planned to correct certain bad features of medical practice; above all, an endeavor will be made to effect better collaboration between directors of clinics and specialists active as consultants.

THE NAZI CREED WITH REGARD TO MEDICINE

The principle address at the inaugural session was delivered by Prof. Franz Hamburger, ordinarius in paediatrics (and successor of Pirquet), long known for his Nazi sympathies. He climaxed his talk with the following pronouncement: "National socialism means a revolution in every sphere of our civilisation and culture. No phase of western culture is unaffected by it. Most noteworthy of all, and what must remain most noteworthy, is the revolution in the realm of medical science, in the field of public health." The speaker went on to say that, despite the achievements of natural science within the past 150 years, medicine had been on the wrong track. "Medicine has now progressed beyond its old frontiers and has broken out of its shell, thanks to the philosophy and deeds of the fuhrer." The healing art of yesterday has become the planned hygiene of today, the medical knowledge of mankind. Thus paediatrics becomes the medical study of children, gynaecology the medical study of women and so on. "With admiral clarity and logic the fuhrer points the way into these fields, "like a physician by the grace of God he shows us the path to health." The rubbish of which physicians must free themselves is the dross of misapplied science, that pseudoscience in medicine which

opposes itself to the clearly ascertainable facts of everyday experience. Hamburger then assailed "that freedom from preconception" which has been such a source of pride. "A real renascence of medical science, on Nazi foundations, must take place." That which is taught by university professors must be completely founded on the tenents of the Nazi program of life and health. "This should be easier for him (the teacher) because national socialism rests on an absolutely sound biological basis." The chief spokesmen of the various medical disciplines at the universities must be confirmed Nazis; this applies especially to clinicians. Hamburger went on to deprecate the "arrogance of physicians" and to put in a good word for "nature medicine," which, he said, ought not to be too lightly esteemed. "National socialism, unlike any other political philosophy or party program, is in accord with the natural history and biology of man. And because national socialism considers all known physiologic data from nature and from human behaviour, it merely represents truths about man. It is accordingly well suited to the direction of the health of our people." Hamburger then turned his fire in succession on Catholicism, liberalism and socialism. He next entered into a discussion of several general problems, in the course of which he said that only a wrongly educated, intellectually biased patient would wish to know the diagnosis-and more along the same line.
JAMA 112 (1939) page 1981

Dr Planner-Plan sets out the political control of science in the new Wiener Medizinsche Gesellschaft. Franz Hamburger shows the direction of this science towards "the clearly ascertainable facts of everyday experience" rather than as he terms it "that dross of misapplied science" from the past. Hans Asperger confirms this approach in the first pages of his paper. "Our method originates in *intuition,* in the attempt to grasp the *structural principle* of the personality." The method of observation as he puts it *"dispenses with a system built according to logical points of view because such a system does not for us appear to correspond to the reality of life".* This method means that the results are not related to logic but rather to the perception of the observer and their view of the "reality of life". This perception is dictated by political ideals rather than by any sound scientific fact. The thing that is wrong is what they think is wrong rather than any physically identifiable abnormality. We don't have faults in chromosomes or identifiable dysfunctions in genes. We have science based on the philosophy of what people should be. At the same time we find that the power of belief far outstretches the limits of conventional science in its appeal to the human psychology. Hans Asperger's work based on Nazi philosophy has proved far more popular than the research we never hear of based on sound scientific principle.

The Nazi ethos with regards to medicine had its origins in the very book that I have at the heart of my own work and that was Darwin's "Origin of Species". Their ideas were based on his notions of natural selection through survival of the fittest. Darwin had pondered for some twenty years as to whether he should publish his work and he had been right to be worried. The fundamental shift away from religious values born out of "The Origin of Species" unleashed science without guidance from religion. His notion of natural selection suffered corruption in the hands of the Social Darwinist movement of the late nineteenth century. "Natural selection" was proposing to become "man made selection" based on the philosophy that natural selection for human beings had effectively ended and so intervention was required to restore balance. Alfred Ploetz was an early proponent of the movement who in 1895 wrote the founding document of what would eventually become the Nazi medical ethos of Racial Hygiene. Ploetz argued that *"if the fit were to be the primary survivors, counter selective forces should be avoided, including medical care for the weak, because this promoted reproduction among them."* (Jeremiah A Barondess, MD Care of the Medical Ethos: Reflections on Social Darwinism, Racial Hygiene and the Holocaust. 1/12/1988 Annals of Internal Medicine Vol 129 issue 11 part 1 pages 891-898.)

The shift away from Christian values in care for the weak would lead to devastating consequences in the Twentieth Century. In 1904 Alfred Ploetz founded the German Society for Racial Hygiene. This organisation promoted the concept of Eugenics in Germany whilst other similar groups promoted the idea of selecting for human beings in Austria, Britain and America. There was a split in Western philosophy after the First World War born out of victory and defeat. German psychology was deeply affected by the country's huge loss of its young men along with its loss of the war. All the deaths had been for nothing and so there was a desire to find purpose from defeat. Into this need stepped the movement in Racial Hygiene. It offered the illusion of the possibility of breeding strength into a defeated people. From this desire for national revitalization we see the Germans pursuing a belief that would lead to their plans for an eventual master race.

Karl Binding and Alfred Hoche, two distinguished German Professors published "The Permission to Destroy Life Unworthy of Life" (Die Freigabe der Vernichtung lebensunwerten Lebens) in 1920. They identified as "unworthy life" incurably ill people along with large segments of the mentally ill, feebleminded and retarded and deformed children. They stressed the therapeutic goal of the concept of destroying life as "purely a healing treatment" and a "healing work". Their views reflected the German mood of the time. Alfred Hoche had lost his own son in the war. It was said that he had been deeply affected by his personal loss along with that of the defeat of the German nation. The bitterness the Germans felt was reflected by the argument that the best young men had died in the war causing a loss to society of the best available genes. The genes of those who did not fight (the worst genes) then proliferated freely, accelerating biological and cultural degeneration. Hoche invoked the concept of "mental death" in various psychiatric conditions and characterised these people as "human ballast." Putting to death "empty shells of human beings" is not to be equated with other types of killings... but [is] an allowable, useful act". *"The Nazi Doctors: Medical Killing and the Psychology of Genocide"*. Dr Robert J Lifton.

Although the concept of direct euthanasia took a little longer to really take off the prevention of future generations of certain sectors of society through sterilisation was embraced quite rapidly. Adolf Hitler recorded his vision in Mein Kamp 1924-1926 in which he stated " *The people's state must see to it that only the healthy beget children...Here the state must act as the guardian of a millennial future...It must put the most modern medical means in the service of this knowledge. It must declare unfit for propagation all who are visibly sick or who have inherited a disease and can therefore pass it on"*.

When the Nazi's took power in Germany in 1933 they quickly enacted laws to prevent the genetically inferior from propagating. The first measure passed on 14th July 1933 was the order of sterilisation of the hereditary sick. The hereditary diseases listed were congenital weak-mindedness, schizophrenia, manic depression, insanity, hereditary epilepsy, hereditary chorea minor, hereditary blindness and deafness, severe hereditary physical deformity and of special importance chronic alcoholism. I have to say it is a good job Hitler didn't come to Britain or the pubs might have shut. The eugenic law was justified in the following words, " *Whereas the families with sound hereditary attributes have, for the most part, adopted the system of one or no children, countless individuals of inferior type and possessing serious hereditary defects are propagating unchecked, with the result that their diseased progeny becomes a burden to society and is threatening, within three generations, to overwhelm completely the valuable strata. Since sterilization is the only sure means of preventing the further hereditary transmission of mental disease and serious defects, this law must be regarded as evidence of brotherly love of watchfulness over the welfare of the coming generation"*. Sterilisation was voluntary under the law that is unless you were in a mental institution or were deemed a violent criminal. In the case of the latter it was proposed that they would be subject to castration under laws to be enacted the following year. The authorities wished make a distinction between sterilisation being a good thing that people should be encouraged to have done and castration being a punishment. JAMA 101 (1933) page 866

The Bavarian commissioner of health, Professor Walter Schultze, gave an indication as to the future in 1933. He declared to the opening ceremony of a state medical facility in Munich his commitment to the use of euthanasia. Schultze stated that *"sterilisation was insufficient: psychopaths, the mentally retarded and other inferior persons must be isolated and killed."* He noted, *"This policy has already been initiated in our concentration camps"*. This statement was significant because it included a group of people that did not fall under the categories listed in the 1933 sterilisation law. There wasn't a clinical diagnosis for the psychopath. Psychopaths could only be identified after they had committed a criminal offence and presumably found themselves in a concentration camp or prison.

The Nazis passed the Law for the Standardisation of the Health System 3rd April 1934, which formed the statutory basis for the creation of a nationwide net of public health offices. They had the purpose of implementing the Nazis program of racial hygiene. At the 1935 Nuremberg Rally Hitler announced his intentions to Gerhard Wagner for the eventual extermination of the handicapped and mentally ill. They were described as "millstone existences" and "useless eaters". By 1940 it is estimated that almost 360,000 people had been sterilised in the German Reich. (The War against the Inferior project by the Documentation Centre of Austrian Resistance Dow)

Shortly after Austria's annexation to Germany in 1938, the Viennese health system began to be restructured on the model of that of Germany's. Dr Planner-Plan and Franz Hamburger's speeches on February 4th 1939 set out the Nazi vision for the future. The public health offices of Vienna underwent a massive expansion. They were in charge of genetic stocktaking in the form of recording genetic and genealogical files. The entire Viennese population was screened for inferior people. The Department for Genetic and Racial Hygiene collected all the incriminating data that was available for mental illnesses, previous venereal diseases, prostitution, alcoholism, hereditary diseases, mental and physical handicaps. In August of 1939 a circular obliged doctors and midwives to report all cases of idiocy and deformities in children to the public health offices. Approximately 700,000 file cards were compiled in all.

Euthanasia

The direct Nazi euthanasia program substantively began outside of concentration camps at the start of the Second World War. Hitler is reported to have thought, by Karl Brandt his personal physician, that the demands and upheavals of war would mute expected religious opposition and enable the euthanasia program to be implemented smoothly. The war effort requires a very healthy people and that the generally diminished sense of the value of human life during war made it " the best time for the elimination of the incurably ill". The first so called "mercy killing or death" occurred on a child named Knauer. He was born blind, with one leg and part of one arm missing and was apparently classified as an "idiot". In late 1938 or early 1939, Hitler ordered Karl Brandt to go to the clinic at the University of Leipzig where the child was being kept to see if the facts were correct and if so then Brandt was to inform the physicians that they could carry out euthanasia in the fuhrer's name and Hitler would quash any potential legal proceedings against them. Karl Brandt reported that the doctors were of the opinion "that there was no justification for keeping [such a child] alive. In his trial at Nuremberg he added that, "it was pointed out that in

128

maternity wards in some circumstances it is quite natural for the doctors themselves to perform euthanasia in such a case without anything further being said about it". To begin with it was the newborns that were killed followed then by the children up to the ages of three or four. After this came the older children followed by adults. At the beginning euthanasia was "kept in a very narrow scope, and to cover only the most serious cases". This would later on become much looser in its criteria and much more extensive.

The first categories for direct euthanasia were set out in a strictly confidential directive (of 18 August 1939) under the pretence "for the clarification of scientific questions in the field of congenital malformation and mental retardation, the earliest possible registration" was required for all children under three where serious hereditary diseases were suspected. These included idiocy, mongolism (especially when associated with blindness and deafness), microcehaly, hydrocephaly, physical malformations, paralysis and spastic conditions. In June 1940 doctors were required to go beyond specific illnesses and conditions and provide in a questionnaire details about birth, elements of family history, especially concerning hereditary illness and such things as excessive use of alcohol, nicotine or drugs, further evaluation of the condition indicating possibilities for improvement, life expectancy, prior institutional observation and treatment, details of physical and mental development and descriptions of convulsions and related phenomena. These questionnaires were then sent to three central medical experts on the Reich Committee for the Scientific Registration of Serious Hereditary and Congenital Ailments who decided which children should be killed. The participating doctors were not made aware of the real reasons for the questionnaires.

The units where the killing was done were parts of children's institutions whose chiefs and prominent doctors were known to be politically reliable and positive towards the goals of the Reich committee. These centres were usually in ordinary clinics and hospitals run by committed Nazis. The children designated to die were dispersed amongst the usual paediatric patients or placed in special wards. In Vienna the Spiegelgrund clinic was the killing centre for those designated for euthanasia. By the end of the war at least 789 children and young people had died there. Some of the children were used for scientific research before being killed. Dr Elmar Turk of the University Children's Clinic used several children for testing a tuberculosis vaccine. Transfer to the killing clinics was achieved by deception through the claim that the children would receive *"under the direction of specialists, all therapeutic possibilities will be administered according to the latest scientific knowledge"*.

Robert J Lifton's book provides us with an insight into the world of the Nazi psychiatrist. He interviewed one who was immediately involved with killing children. This is what the doctor had to say *" According to the thinking of that time, in the case of children killing seemed somehow justifiable...whereas in the case of the adult mentally ill, that was definitely pure murder"* He described an interaction between the child-victim without ordinary human feelings. *"whom one cannot speak to, who does not laugh, who affectively unapproachable such an executioner does not have that bad feelings...there is a lack of affective tension, the emotional participation...and that can turn any human being into a murderer."* Another physician explained how the killing was done and how it was explained to parents. *" A very excitable child completely idiotic....could not be kept quiet with the normal dose of sedatives,"* so that *"an overdose....had to be used in order to....avoid endangering itself through its own restlessness."* At the same time *"we physicians know that such an overdose of a sedative, for children usually luminal....could cause pneumonia,...and that is virtually incurable."* This is how the killing was done. Luminal tablets were dissolved in liquid and given to the condemned child to drink. The sedative was given repeatedly morning and night over two or three days until the child lapsed into a continuous sleep. Pneumonia would set in and be the final cause of death. If the children developed a tolerance to the usual sedative because they had been given so much of it a fatal dose of morphine-scopolamine could be given to achieve the same effect. These children were killed under the "diagnosis useless".

The Psychopath

We commonly associate the term psychopath with mass murderers and the like however this is a bit of a misconception. The dictionary definition of the term is "A person with a personality disorder, especially one manifested in aggressively antisocial behaviour, amoral attitudes, and continually fluctuating moods." Nazi ideology required children as well as adults to conform to the regimes radical expectations of obedience, discipline and the performance and hatred of the supposedly inferior people. The model child was active, physically fit and a disciplined conformist. These children had to be deliberately differentiated from the "romantic", "awkwardly intellectual" and the "socialist revolutionary type". This is how the new order viewed the previous supposedly weak rulers of Germany that took up power after the First World War. Hitler set out his vision for the youth of the Reich in the following words *"My program for educating youth is hard. Weakness must be hammered away. In my castles of Teutonic Order a youth will grow up before which the world will tremble. I want a brutal, domineering, fearless, cruel youth. Youth must be all that. It must bear pain. There must be nothing weak and gentle about it. The free splendid beast of prey must once again flash from its eyes... That is how I will eradicate thousands of years of human domestication... That is how I will create the New Order".* This vision was one of mass killers trained and functioning together under the control of the Reich. These children obediently conformed to nazi doctrine and unquestioningly worshiped the furher and his vision. In October 1932 70,000 such youngsters crammed into a stadium at Potsdam in Germany. This was a movement on mass of children indoctrinated with nazi ideology. There was no place in Hitler's Reich for the non-conformist. (Hitler's Children) by Guido Knopp.

In 1937 The Vienna Psychiatric and Neurologic Association appointed a committee to study the problem of revised insanity laws for Austria. Prominent in the legislative program sponsored by this group was the establishment of state detention institutions for psychopaths who, although not insane within the legal definition, were nevertheless a public menace. Professor Berze pointed out in a lecture to the association that among the psychopaths of the "borderline" type who, in the absence of any definitive mental disease, cannot be declared "insane" are recruited those mentally subnormal criminals who constitute a permanent social menace. If one of these persons is convicted of an offence he may perhaps receive a light punishment or be placed under observation in a psychiatric institution for a time, then soon released as "not insane" to prey upon society. And this occurs even if the person presents an obvious picture of moral insanity. Under the existing Austrian law it is impossible to keep a criminal of the "borderline" type in permanent detention as the hospitals for the insane were already filled to capacity with genuine mental cases. The Vienna psychiatrists recommended not only the detention of dangerous psychopaths but a continuous systematic supervision of all psychopathic persons. This would assure special legal protection of the non-criminal psychopaths. Any abnormal person who believes that some one has wronged or offended him who accordingly utters threats, can, under the proposed legislation, be rendered harmless before he has had the time to make good his threats. (JAMA 109, 1937 page 1465)

In 1939 The Society of German Neurologists and Psychiatrists met in Wiesbaden. The president, Professor Rudin, pointed out that psychiatry in its efforts for improving racial hygiene performed a timely and progressive service. He accredited psychiatry with having been the first division of medicine to point out to the state and the national socialist party the dangers latent in psychopathic persons and to give impetus to the well-known legal measures taken. It was fallacious to assume, he said, that psychiatry would become increasingly superfluous, because psychopaths according to the laws governing racial hygiene would soon die out. This assumption involves the danger of deterioration for the psychiatric profession, whereas psychiatry requires the most competent physicians, because it deals with many dangerously ill with hereditary psychoses. He said, "The individual therapeutist may bungle and mar one or two human lives, but the poor psychiatrist, whole generations". Rudin warned against undermining the reputation of psychiatrists. It would seem there was a bit of job protectionism going on here and a bit of a worry that all their clients would soon be dead and they would be out of work. (JAMA 113 1939 page 1501)

The problem with the 1937 proposal for revision of the insanity laws in Austria was how to identify a "borderline" psychopath. In 1939 we can see the psychiatry profession congratulating itself for its part in efforts to eliminate these people. However only the psychopaths that had committed offences and had been caught must have been subject to sterilisation or worse. The ones that hadn't been caught for offences were neither in concentration camps nor mental institutions. They weren't clinically diagnosable because there wasn't a recognised category for clinical diagnosis. As was pointed out in 1937 "The hospitals for the insane were already full of genuine mental cases". They couldn't, as things stood, be identified for the latent dangers they supposedly posed to society and racial hygiene. The proposal for the continuous systematic monitoring of all psychopathic persons couldn't be implemented either to protect the non-criminal element or neutralise the others. In 1943 Hans Asperger published his paper setting out a typology for identifying autistic psychopaths in childhood.

Uta Frith in her book "Autism and Asperger Syndrome" sets out Hans Asperger's observations of the class of children he was studying, which culminated in his diagnosis and categorisation on publication of his paper entitled "Die "Autitischen Psychopathen" im Kindesalter" 1943. The question arises as to what would be the fate of these children. Looking at Asperger's case studies he is very matter of fact about his observations. He records what he sees and what he is told. In accordance with nazi directives he provides family histories, prior institutional observation and treatment, details of birth along with possibilities for improvement. This took the form remedial pedagogy with treatment falling within medical rather than educational jurisdiction.

To fit in with the diagnosis of a "psychopath" in accordance with the dictionary definition we do need an element of "aggressive antisocial behaviour". Asperger records in his case studies as follows: For the first child listed "He quickly became aggressive and lashed out with anything he could get hold of (once a hammer), regardless of the danger to others....He had attacked other children". In the second case Asperger records "One of the principle reasons for his being referred by the school was his savage tendency to fight. Little things drove him to senseless fury, whereupon he attacked other children, gnashing his teeth and hitting out blindly. This was dangerous because he was not a skilled fighter. Children who are skilled fighters know exactly how far they can go and can control their movements so that they hardly ever cause real trouble." In the third case we have "He was never able to get on with other children. It was impossible to go to the park with him, as he would instantly get embroiled in fighting. Apparently, he hit or verbally abused other children indiscriminately." Only in the fourth case do we depart from the aggressive behaviour and so things might be getting better you might say? Well perhaps not this child was too fat to fight. Asperger describes him "His appearance was grotesque. On top of a massive body, over the big face with flabby cheeks, was a tiny skull." "It was not surprising, then, that he was continuously taunted by other children who ran after him in the street. Of course, he could never do anything to his fleet-footed tormentors, becoming only more ridiculous in his helpless rage." Asperger further describes him as "an autistic automaton" and considers "his autism was due to a brain injury at birth." This final case study is a particularly short one. We might suspect that this type of boy is straight off for some luminal medication under a previous category. It would seem from the descriptions provided by the doctors previously that the children who were properly autistic had already gone under the category "idiotic".

Most of the nazi requirements were missing in the children Asperger studied. They did not conform to authority as required by complete obedience to the fuhrer. They were not physically well coordinated as required by the Nazi obsession for physically fit people. They did not function as part of a group as required by Nazi doctrine where everybody functioned solely for the interests of the Nazi state. Their intellectual abilities were not especially of value and were in fact resented in some ways as hallmarks of the old order in the form of the "awkwardly intellectual". On the face of it these children had no saving graces in the Third Reich.

Nazi goals were directed towards the value of human life to the state. The seriously disabled, Jews and Gypsies were deemed to have no value and so were put to death. The psychopaths however firstly needed to be identified and then distinguished between for the criminal and none criminal types if the 1937 Austrian proposals were to establish their value. Asperger stresses the positive value of this personality in the working world by stating that they had found a "large number of" such "people whose mathematical ability determines their professions: mathematics, technologists, industrial chemists and high-ranking civil servants." At the same time he describes spiteful and malicious behaviour in the children he observed, which would point one might think towards criminality. He feels that further comparison is required with works by other authors characterising personality types and postpones any real definitive conclusion. He states that the "debate will undoubtedly become more fruitful when we know what becomes of our autistic children when they are adults. This awaits a later comprehensive study".

The question we need to ask is why actually create a mental disorder and then try and defend it by stating its positive value in the working world? It would make more sense not to call these people mentally disordered at all? I think this goes back to the 1937 Austrian proposals for the continuous systematic supervision of all psychopathic persons. Translation of the first pages of Asperger's paper reveals that the lead term he is using is psychopath. This features early on with autistic arising towards the end. The use of the term autistic is merely incidental to the main description that Asperger is creating. This gives some illusion of mental disorder in order that the psychopath may be classified with a clinical category for monitoring. The next question is where is the easiest place to find all potential psychopaths? The answer is in school because it is the one place pretty much everybody can be found. After people leave school they disperse into the working world and are virtually impossible to monitor on a systematic basis. Is this is why we have autistic psychopathy in childhood? Asperger doesn't know the outcome for the children he studied and whether they will turn into criminal psychopaths or not. This is why he considers that a definitive conclusion awaits a later comprehensive study when his subjects become adults. This study never happened and for good reason. This is because it is virtually impossible to identify who will become a psychopath in the criminal sense. Efforts to do so would be futile because criminality is born out of circumstance not psychology. Asperger's children would have likely revealed nothing of any consequence as far as criminality is concerned had they been seen as adults.

Hans Asperger kept his work very sensibly quiet to the outside world until just before he died. As well as autistic psychopathy he also wrote papers on the subject of death. In the Third Reich death was deeply ingrained in Nazi ideology. At an ancient Germanic site in Murnau in Upper Bavaria there was a memorial decked in the symbols of the Reich with the slogan "We were born to die for Germany". Nazi indoctrination meant that "You are nothing, your Volk (state) is everything." To die for the Furher and the Volk was the greatest honour of all. Just before the fall of Berlin at the end of the war Carl Diem gave a fiery speech to young people at the site of the 1936 Berlin Olympics. He held up the young people as the shining example of the tiny band of Spartans fighting to the death against the Persians at Thermopylae: "Death is a fine thing when the noble warrior falls for the Fatherland."

The question we need to ask ourselves is if Asperger's work has such a dubious origin how has it found its way into modern day psychology? The answer to this is not clear. Uta Frith does claim in her book to have a dash of autism herself. If this is the case then there can be a naivety that goes with the autistic mind where it believes what it is being told is true. Because this mind is naturally honest it doesn't always understand that other people use honesty in a beneficial fashion to themselves and do not always tell the full truth in context. She failed to provide a translation of the first pages of Asperger's paper in her book. It is in these pages that the National Socialist scientific basis for the research is set out under the method of observation used which, as Asperger puts it, *"dispenses with a system built according to logical points of view because such a system does not for us appear to correspond to the reality of life"*

There is a more sinister perspective we need to consider and this is the possible rise of National Socialism once again. The potential for this is not in Germany or Austria but is here in Britain. The rebirth of Asperger's classification on mass also coincides with a period of socialism in this country. However what does it take for socialism to become National Socialism. This happens when the state's welfare takes precedence over the rights of the individuals in it. It happens when a council's welfare takes precedence over the rights of the taxpayer complaining about it. It happens when a school's welfare takes precedence over the rights of the children and parents using it. In these circumstances we are starting to look at the beginnings of a Nazi state. We are fed with plots by terrorists, which may be true. However the government make the most of it for implementing their surveillance society. Islamic women in veils are identified as threats because they don't show their faces to confirm they are who they say they are on their bus passes. In two years time all our children's records are planned to go on a national database in the interests of child protection. This is remarkably similar to what has gone before with the 700,000 file cards compiled in Vienna in the interests of protecting the health of the Reich. How can we be sure that the records will not be used for systematic discrimination against the so defined undesirables? The man in charge of protecting our personal information recognises this potential problem. In the Times dated 28th October 2006 the Information Commissioner is recorded as saying "We're waking up in a surveillance society" "and when you start to see how many well-intentioned, apparently beneficial schemes are in place to monitor people's activities and movements, I think that does raise concerns. It can stigmatise people. I have worries about technology being used to identify classes of people who present some sort of risk to society."

On 5th November 2006 I found an incredible article on the front page of the Sunday Times, which took me right back to 1939. However this is not a historical article it is a current one. The Royal College of Obstetricians and Gynaecology is calling on the health profession to consider permitting euthanasia of seriously disabled newborn babies. The college is arguing that "active euthanasia" should be considered for the overall good of families, to spare parents the emotional burden and financial hardship of bringing up the sickest babies. In the article it says that the college states "A very disabled child can mean a disabled family". Dr Pieter Sauer, co-author of Groningen, which is the Dutch national guidelines for legal euthanasia in Holland, claims that British paediatricians already perform mercy killings, and says the practice should be open. Worse still however John Harris, a member of the government's Human Genetics Commission welcomed the college's views. He is stated as saying "We can terminate for serious foetal abnormality up to term but cannot kill a newborn. What do people think is happening down the birth canal to make it okay to kill the foetus at one end of the birth canal but not at the other". Perhaps it is not right to kill at either end of the birth canal. The article finishes by stating "The cost of treating very premature babies is high. A neonatal intensive care bed costs about £1000 a day and extremely premature babies can require intensive care for four months". Are we again looking at the prospect of killing "useless eaters", "millstone existences" and "human ballast".

On 27th November 2006 I read in the Times that the police are targeting dangerous suspects before they can offend. Laura Richards, a senior criminal psychologist with the Homicide Prevention Unit, told the Times "My vision is that we know across London who the top 100 people are. We need to know who we are targeting." "It is trying to pick up Ian Huntley before he goes out and commits that murder. Then we have the opportunity to stop something turning into a lethal event". This sounds rather familiar to what happened in the Third Reich with the targeting of psychopaths for sterilisation or worse. Now I am aware of three murders that have involved alleged Asperger's Syndrome. I am not saying that all people with the label will be murderers, in just the same way as I wouldn't say all black people will be involved in drive by shootings, far from it in fact. However if our society is going to adopt National Socialist values and arrest people before they do anything I would suggest it would be a good idea to lose the label before its too late.

There is a poem that I feel is most appropriate when considering the values a society should adopt. This poem came from experiences in the Nazi Third Reich.

First they came for the communists and I did not speak out because I was not a Communist.

Then they came for the Socialists and I did not speak out because I was not a Socialist.

Then they came for the trade unionists and I did not speak out because I was not a trade unionist.

Then they came for the Jews and I did not speak out because I was not a Jew.

Then they came for me and there was no one left to speak out for me.

Pastor Niemoller

The point of the poem is that under National Socialist doctrine the Knauer child was perhaps the beginning however once it starts when is it to be the turn of your child? Under such doctrine any non-conformist opposition is expelled. Would you be expelled? Non-conformists are essential in civilised society to keep it functioning. There has to be opposition to authority to prevent the state from going too far. Everybody has to be kept because once the weakest person has been removed there is always another weakest to replace them and then they have to be removed. Just as in the tribe compassion needs to prevent this from happening for without it society would eventually be reduced to a single person.

I do recognise the argument that Asperger's Syndrome is useful in trying to protect children from exclusion from school and persecution. The fault however really lies with the management of our schools rather than with the children themselves. When we think about it there isn't any real management. Decisions are taken by school governors who are at the bottom level of the democratic decision making process. County councils are the next level up and they push the value of local democracy close to the point of worthless. Protection needs to be made possible without a dubious label of mental disorder. My favoured approach would be to allow all people free access to a discrimination tribunal based on the violation of basic human rights. There should be no need to be classified with a dubious disability to get access to affordable justice.

Most fundamentally when we consider the origin of "Autistic Psychopathy" there has to be real doubt cast on Hans Asperger's classification of a mental disorder. The whole basis for Asperger's Syndrome is likely to be wrong. That is the case unless you believe in Nazi doctrine. Rather than him observing a disorder in human personality traits he was actually observing behaviour that was perfectly normal just not perhaps completely desirable in the Reich.

Chapter Sixteen

Observation of the characteristics of the original mind

Diagnosis of Asperger's Syndrome is achieved through identifying what is termed a triad of impairments in socialisation, communication and imagination. These impairments are relative to the tribal mind and reflect a lack of inherited ability from evolution. As far as socialisation and communication is concerned this arises from not evolving to naturally socialise and in turn communicate with other people. The lack of imagination is actually a reflection of a lack of natural ability with stories rather than imagination as such. This mind did not evolve to recreate and conceptualise stories. They came from the tribe and were originally for entertainment. What is often perceived as a profound problem is actually quite trivial in reality.

I will take you through a more detailed list of characteristics that are presently used to identify what is termed Asperger's Syndrome. These characteristics are underlined and taken from the Internet in 2004. I will provide my explanation for the characteristics from evolution.

I do apologise if I seem to keep repeating myself but I do want you to see just how clearly the evolutionary model I have set out is justified by the characteristics of this classified disorder. Further more I want you to see how our evolutionary story shows these characteristics to be normal.

Social characteristics

Difficulty in accepting criticism or correction: That's because I'm right! The original man never had anybody to

142

tell him what to do. In the tribe he had a special place and was the one doing the telling. In evolution the original mind was not criticised because there was no one to criticise it. There is therefore no naturally programmed reaction to criticism. This mind functions in a "single minded fashion" and this very term means without thought to what other people may be thinking. The tribal mind had to evolve to accept criticism because it was inevitable at some time or other when living in a group. Even the chief would get it in fact he probably got more of it than most. Without a natural ability to accept criticism the tribe would not function. The chief and his people would be too busy sulking or hitting each other to get on with the business of tribal life.

Difficulty in offering correction or criticism without appearing harsh, pedantic or insensitive: The original man never developed a natural understanding of the social-niceties necessary in the tribe to stop unnecessary fights between tribal members. Humour naturally evolved in the tribal mind to deal with and pass criticism. Offence is avoided in using a joke but the criticism is still made. Laughing at the joke although perhaps with gritted teeth helps diffuse the offence in the person who is the butt of the joke. Furthermore the original mind is naturally honest. This means there will tend to be a more honest approach, which doesn't always sit well with the way the tribe, would say things. In the tribe the "white lie" evolved to avoid creating upset between members. This dishonesty served a natural evolutionary purpose in ensuring the tribe could function together as a group.

Difficulty in perceiving and applying unwritten social rules or protocols: These rules only ever existed in the tribe as a necessary way of maintaining order. They are natural to the tribal mind. For instance it would be unseemly to go up to the chief and tell him he was a complete idiot in thinking that it was a good idea to try and catch a three-ton rhinoceros for dinner. There were the chief's sensitivities to think of plus the fact you would get a good clobbering.

Naturally evolved social etiquette in the tribe precluded this kind of behaviour. Those that didn't evolve etiquette found themselves booted out with consequently a rather bleak prospect of survival. The original family never needed etiquette or developed a natural understanding of these tribal social rules. It's interesting that the word etiquette is derived from French rather than Anglo Saxon English. French society is more geared towards tribal behaviour than is British society. We have evolved expressions such as "f_ck off" which I think says it all about the minds that originally formed England.

Immature Manners: The original family didn't have manners. Manners only existed in the tribe to avoid tribal members upsetting each other. Manners are quite complex and extend into most areas of tribal behaviour. There are eating manners for instance and this particularly means not eating with your mouth open but also not gobbling food. In the tribe everybody had to share the food and it was not a free for all. There was structure to the eating in order that the chief got the best bits as reward for his position but also to ensure that each member got their fair share. There are manners in conversation. For instance it is not polite to cut people off in mid sentence however if the sentence is an hour long it can be tempting but still uncomfortable. There are manners in greetings and departures. All these manners served to create social cohesion in the tribe. In the original family natural manners never evolved because there was simply no evolutionary purpose to them.

Naïve trust in others: The original man was only ever honest. Dishonesty could only exist between two people and came with the spoken word which evolved in the tribe. As far as the original family is concerned there is only what is and what is not. With the concept of dishonesty comes the counterbalancing concept of trust. In the tribal mind there is a natural caution over trust because of the existence of lies. For the original mind this natural caution has not evolved for there were no lies in the original single-family existence. The difference between the tribal and original mind with regards to honesty is reflected in the cultures of different countries. Those where the original mind is more dominant are inherently more honest. It is this honesty that facilitates business and growth.

Shyness: Shyness served the purpose of separating people in the original desert existence. Because people developed a natural shyness they spread out over the land and this increased the foraging area for each family. The families that weren't shy and stayed close to other families would not survive this period in evolution and would die out through lack of food. Shyness served an essential evolutionary purpose at man's most critical point in the battle for survival. In the tribe shyness was watered down so that people could function together as a group. People needed to be relatively unafraid of each other for the tribe to work efficiently.

Low or no conversational participation in group meetings or conferences: The original mind only took part in meetings after the substantive end of natural selection of mental characteristics for this basic mind type. Therefore there is no natural understanding of how meetings should operate. For the original mind there is only the telling to the meeting of what should be and what should not be as far as it is concerned. Meetings themselves serve the purpose of confirming status within the tribe. The chief needs to demonstrate his authority so everybody knows he's still the chief. If you think about a typical meeting how much is usually achieved? In my experience not a great deal. They are useful for disseminating information provided people don't nod off. Decisions and agreements come down to one or two people making them or agreeing them. Even in a committee we tend to find only one or two decision makers with the rest just going along.

Constant anxiety about performance and acceptance, despite recognition and commendation: The original family didn't stop in the original existence in the desert until it went to sleep. The obsessive search for food was what ensured survival. Even if hunger was satisfied, and that was rare, the search continued to accumulate food in case the next day was less succesful. This behaviour formed the basis of what would develop into capitalism and the acquisition of assets for future benefit. There is no real end point in this behaviour for there is always more to be acquired. Success can be measured on a never-ending scale. Something can always be better.

In the tribe the mind would evolve a different form of behaviour. Other people's commendation of your efforts or status would give satisfaction and this pleasure served to bond and motivate the group. For the original mind status and commendation are not a natural concept it understands. There were no other people in the original existence to gain status in front of or commendation from.

There is a characteristic that is born out of this behaviour and that is the characteristic of the perfectionist. Because something can always be better in the eyes of the original mind it doesn't reach that point of satisfaction. This is an essential ingredient in creativity particularly in the case of the most extraordinary achievements.

<u>Scrupulous honesty, often expressed in an apparently disarming or inappropriate manner or setting</u>: Dishonesty only existed between two people in the tribe. There were certain degrees of honesty that didn't serve a natural positive purpose. For instance telling the chief he was no good in bed would not ingratiate you into his affections if you were a woman aspiring to high status in the tribe.

Tribal people evolved to use honesty in a way that was beneficial to themselves and to the tribe as a whole. The original mind didn't evolve in this way. It is naturally honest and lacks the natural evolutionary development of the tribal mind to use honesty in a beneficial fashion. This means that honesty expressed by the original mind can appear inappropriate at times. For instance telling someone they are fat doesn't serve a beneficial purpose to the original mind or to the person who is fat. A fat person is most likely to know that for themselves and the original mind making this choice observation is likely to get a thick ear.

Bluntness in emotional expression: Most of emotion comes from the tribal existence. These emotions were necessary for the tribe to function. The original single-family existence in the desert life was not easy but extremely simple. There was the obsessive search for food and not a lot else. Finding a sexual partner was simple due to a lack of choice that's if you could find one at all. There was no chatting up to be done for there was no language. When you did find a girl it didn't take a great deal to impress her. In fact finding her at all was probably quite impressive in its self and showed you were at least good at walking. The original boy would have demonstrated his affections by taking her out to dinner. She would want to see if you were able to find food, as that was what mattered and not a lot else.

Discomfort manipulating or playing games with others: The original family never played games apart from with the children as a teaching experience for life. There were no other people to manipulate in the original way of life. Manipulation is in effect selling to them be it an idea or an item. This behaviour stems from the tribe and was formed by the need to get other tribal members to do what one tribal member thought seemed like a good idea.

The usual sales patter would come from the chief. He would come up with a good idea for the hunt and need to sell it to a sceptical tribe. This required manipulation particularly if the idea wasn't really a very good one at all. He would need to manipulate the men's feeling of loyalty. They couldn't be loyal if they weren't brave enough to catch the three-ton rhinoceros. Just think of the poor hungry children and the contempt that the women would feel if you didn't do this little thing for them. I am sure the women will make it more than worth your while when you get back, well have an orgy that will be nice.

One of the defining characteristics of the autistic personality, which can be seen in early childhood, is a lack of imaginative play. This is a little misleading because we are not actually observing a lack of imagination as such but rather a lack of imagination expressed in the recreation of stories. There is no inherited interest in stories in the original mind because stories evolved in the tribe with the spoken word. This mind is naturally interested in things it can see as fact rather than the stories it is told.

Un-modulated reaction in being manipulated patronized or handled by others: The original family lived alone and there is no natural understanding of being sold to or being handled by other people. The very act of being sold to requires a degree of gullibility. Gullibility evolved in the tribe. The men would take on board the chief's idea for the rhino hunt and think that sounds like a good idea but would not be altogether sure. As for the original mind it does not like being controlled by other people. It has evolved to think for itself and not to be told what to think. The reaction to being told what to think or do can be excessive in the event that self-control hasn't been instilled by learnt behaviour.

As for being physically handled this again evolved in the tribe and helped with bonding. Expressions of group pleasure would involve hugging and other such physical contact. For the original mind there was no physical contact. This mind is also more sensitive to touch and so a normal grasp of the arm can feel painful. This in turn induces fear with a consequent lashing out for the purpose of getting away.

Low to medium level of paranoia: The CIA will get me for this - well perhaps not. The tendency to be paranoid could well be inherited in so far as it might motivate effort to find

148

food in a harsh environment with the fear of hunger the motivating force. When caring for the flock it serves the purpose of always being on your guard on the look out for predators and stray animals. Paranoia could also have been selected for naturally later in evolution when we will see original minds hiding away in the remote locations, which will be dealt with in the next chapter of our story. I would suspect that paranoia is in part inherited; however a portion of it is acquired through learnt behaviour.

Children do not tend to show paranoia unless they have been through negative experiences. For the original mind the opportunity to acquire negative experiences is greatly increased in social situations. The typical problem faced is that of being bullied in school. Bullying is a natural basic animal instinct, which occurs in a group and is likely to arise from our existence in the trees. In the tribe we see bullying in the form of the gang. Both the original and tribal minds have inherited the natural ability to bully. As for the bullied, with an excess of negative experience comes paranoia that more bad things will happen.

The irrational nature of some of the paranoid fears is born out of the original mind's ability to convince itself something is true. We see a fear that the government is out to get you. Then again maybe they are. The Holocaust would have selected for the paranoid as it would be these people that would have escaped and lived to reproduce. In the tribe we see confidence gained from herd mentality. Just as in a flock of sheep the individual animal gains confidence from the fact it is unlikely that particular animal will be killed. The same was true in the tribe. Chances were that it was going to be somebody else that was going to get it not you.

Low to no apparent sense of humour: Humour evolved in the tribe to avoid unnecessary conflict between tribal members. They naturally developed language and hence jokes. Jokes served the purpose of making a point without offending another tribal member. Humour is also learnt

149

through dealing with trauma. Tribal minds have a natural level of humour however it is the original mind living through trauma that can take humour to outstanding levels. This behaviour is learnt and helps the mind to cope with the traumatic events that are being experienced. Trauma is a chance event dependant on circumstance and so there is the opportunity for no humour to be acquired. This perhaps requires a little qualification in so far as if there is any humour present it isn't apparent to anybody else.

The original mind more naturally understands the humour of observing funny behaviour rather than jokes. It better understands slap-stick comedy_ which is the first mass manufactured form of humour. We see the likes of Chaplin and Laural and Hardy producing the earliest film comedy based on this form of original humour. The pure joke telling comedian came later and was popular for a time when I was a child although not anymore. Today we see a combination of the two in the form situation comedy.

Difficulty with reciprocal displays of pleasantries and greetings: I tell you I wish the bloke that wrote this stuff would just get on with it. The original man didn't have patience and he didn't need it. He never had to wait for another man to tell him what to do. Pleasantries and greetings serve the purpose of creating ease between tribal people. The tribe would on occasion meet up with other tribes and this was a necessary process to prevent excessive inbreeding. Girls and perhaps boys would be swapped between tribes to spread the gene pool.

The tribal mind evolved to have the ability of interaction with other tribes. Greetings served the purpose gaining trust with people who were not regularly seen. The handshake is known as an indicator that there is no concealed knife in the hand. Pleasantries serve the purpose of creating ease particularly prior to negotiations. The original mind in the original existence evolved to keep out of the way of other people. Meetings were counter-productive to survival for they meant people were too close together. The original mind didn't evolve a natural ability for having contact with other people.

Problems expressing empathy or comfort with others: sadness condolence, congratulations etc: There is no compassion in the original man's world apart from for the family. There were no other people to care about. In the tribe there were other people to care about and empathy evolved to make the tribe function as a group. They cared for and had compassion for each other. If somebody died everybody in the tribe would feel the hurt. This served the evolutionary purpose of making the tribe look after one and other. The feeling of loss and grief served to enhance effort in keeping everybody alive which, in turn, enhanced the tribe's prospect of survival. This goes back to the basic principle that if only the strongest was kept this would lead to a single man and the tribe could not naturally function.

Difficulty with adopting a social mask to obscure real feelings, moods, and reactions: The original family did not live a social existence and hence never evolved a natural social mask to obscure real feelings. In the tribe it was on occasion necessary to keep ones true feelings to one's self for the good of relationships within the tribe. For instance displeasure at one of the chief's especially daft ideas was better hidden because he was particularly good at painful arm locks and ear twists. So we see a natural ability evolve in the tribal mind to hide feelings that are counter productive to the functioning of the group.

Abrupt and strong expression of likes and dislikes: The original man was naturally honest and things either were or they were not. He either liked things or he didn't. As part of a social group in the tribe people had different likes and dislikes. The tribe however has to function as one and so moderation of these likes and dislikes was necessary for social cohesion. Compromise had to be found in behaviour so that the group could function together.

Rigid adherence to rules and social conventions where flexibility is desirable: The very existence of strict discipline originates from the original mind. These strict disciplines allowed original minds to function together in the creation of civilisation and I am going to tell you how that happened in the next chapter. The modern world has reached a level of such complexity in an attempt to maintain discipline that rules have started to become counter productive. There can be too many rules and people start to ignore them. Flexibility is a desirable feature, as nobody likes a "job's worth". However the point at which flexibility becomes taking no notice of the rules is always a difficult line to draw.

It is also worth pointing out that the original mind is naturally less flexible in its nature. It evolved to survive by constantly searching for food with little variation from the daily routine. The tribal mind evolved greater flexibility through variation of routine borne out of life in the tribe.

Apparent absence of relaxation, recreational, or time out activities: The original family didn't stop and neither should its descendants. In the original existence survival was ensured only by the constant search for food. Only those minds that kept constantly on the go survived. Recreation is a tribal concept as only the tribe had time for recreation. The tribal existence was more successful than the original existence in the desert by virtue of the improved environmental conditions of the time. Large kills lasted a few days and there was plenty more bison to kill another day. The tribe evolved to enjoy recreation, which in its turn enhanced pleasure in the tribal existence through increased enjoyment. Only the tribal mind has inherited this natural concept.

Known for single-mindedness: The original man had to be focussed to succeed and this evolved from the simple business of following animal tracks. There was the female mind in this existence but this mind had the separate function of searching widely for food that could be seen in the present. Although the two depended on each other for survival they didn't consciously cooperate as such for the majority of the time. Each had its innate natural purpose selected for by evolution. In the modern day the existence of language can upset this natural balance particularly when it's in the hands of the wife. In the original existence there were no such unpleasant complications.

Flash Temper: There was no need for patience with other people in the original existence in the desert because there weren't any at least not ones that were met very often. The flash temper could even have helped serve the purpose of evolutionary survival. On the odd occasion that people strayed into other people's territory the unrestrained display of gesticulation soon solved the problem. In the tribe temper needed to be restrained for the purposes of social adhesion. Still the occasional rant by the chief was not unknown particularly when you had done something especially stupid.

Tantrums: The original man always got his own way and so should his child. Not that mine does because that would mean I wouldn't and we couldn't have that. The tantrum is one of the classical problems encountered with the original mind. What we see here is a battle of wills. Both parties want their own way because they have both inherited that desire. It is crucial from the beginning that the parent imposes its will. This requires substantial effort because in effect the parent is battling against his or her own personality. The child has inherited part of this personality and he or she can have greater energy and less distraction in the pursuit of personal desires. Should the final conflict come down to the simple matter of size then the parent has lost the battle. As a matter of self-respect this cannot be. The child's time for winning will come all in good time when the parent is well out of the way.

Excessive talk: This comes from the full range of language ability available to the original mind. This can equally be very little talk. All language is learnt by this mind and there is no natural understanding of it. The original mind doesn't like listening and much prefers talking. The original man didn't listen to anybody. This can make teaching rather difficult and stubborn behaviour requires modification in order that necessary information can be imparted. There is one lesson that the original mind really needs to learn. This is to listen to what it is told. The drip-drip effect can be useful with the especially stubborn. The idea can be planted and allowed to grow. The mind then eventually thinks it is its own idea and then all is well.

Difficulty in forming friendships and intimate relationships: Friendship predates the original-single family existence and wasn't based on cooperative behaviour. It was based on the pleasure of the company of friends. When you think about these relationships between adults today they have the characteristic of occasional or regular meetings of friends but the relationship is not one of living together. In the original single-family existence there were no friends. There is however some ability in the original mind to form friendships particularly on a family sized scale. Difficulty arises in finding two compatible people. It has to be born in mind that each original mind likes to do its own thing and compromise is not a natural feature. Friends are necessary in school and at the time a girl friend or boy friend needs to be found. These relationships provide protection and were the very start of the tribe. As far as love is concerned the conventional view is tribal. The original version is simpler perhaps less intense but longer lasting. Again it is a question of compatibility, which is not as easy to achieve as it is for the tribal mind.

Social isolation and intense concern for privacy: The original family lived in isolation and isolation was essential for survival in the desert. The original mind today should prefer isolation just as it did in the past. It is the tribal mind that likes to be part of a group. It feels safe and enjoys the benefits of tribal group behaviour.

Limited clothing preference discomfort with formal attire or uniforms: This is probably because this clobber is uncomfortable, stiff and prickly. Uniforms are designed for tribal minds, which aren't as sensitive to discomfort. The very concept of uniform is for someone who is told what to do and to signify status in the form of rank. Original minds are the ones that excel in whatever field they find suits their interests. Recognition of this is the adoption of a more personalised uniform for these people. In the police senior detectives are allowed to wear their own suits. The existence of uncomfortable uniforms does serve to preclude some of the most capable people from some of the services that require them most.

Preference for bland or bare environments in living arrangements: In the original way of life the original family didn't have a house. They roamed their territory and by necessity travelled light. They only carried what they needed. Adornments were part of tribal living and signified status. The more painful the adornment, the tougher the tribal man, hence the higher his status in the tribe. These adornments are still used on the body in the form of body piercing and tattoos and jewellery. Adornments are also used on cars and in the home to signify status. The original mind isn't intuitively aware of status and is also more sensitive to pain hence it is less likely to go for personal adornments. Equally it shouldn't naturally be into adornments on cars or in the home.

Difficulty judging others personal space: The original family wasn't physically close to other people. Only in the tribe did people live close together and a natural understanding of personal space became a necessity for tribal living. This can reflect itself in standing too close or too far away from another person.

Limited by intensely pursued interests: The original man was highly focused and obsessive. He had to be to survive. Food was scarce and it was only by obsessive searching that enough could be found to live on. Those that didn't

155

search obsessively died. The original mind still has the same obsessive make up which is expressed in different ways in modern life. This expression can be in a single interest for a long period of time or different interests for shorter periods of time. The common theme will be one interest at a time and a high degree of focus. It is the obsessive characteristics of the original mind that is the key to exceptional performance. All genius is created by obsession. The adage of 5% inspiration and 95% perspiration is true of genius and reflects the importance of obsession in achievement.

Often perceived as being in their own world: This is simply a reflection of higher level of focus in the original mind. This focus evolved out of following tracks of animals in the obsessive search for food. To achieve this focus extraneous factors are shut out. Hence it is likely that the original mind wont hear what other people are saying unless it fits in with what the original mind is thinking about at the time. This is at least my excuse to the wife anyway. The tribal mind evolved to take account of the people around it for it was cooperative behaviour that ensured survival in the tribe.

Physical manifestations

Strong sensory sensitivities touch, sounds, vision and smell: The original man was more sensitive and so is the original mind. This level of sensitivity varies with the level of activity of the mind. It was in the tribe that the senses were reduced in their intensity as cooperative behaviour became more important than acute senses. What we are observing is the relative difference.

Uncomfortable clothing can be an issue to the original mind. Noise pollution may be a problem. Light pollution may affect it more and smells could be an issue that it notices. When the original man existed all these senses would be used to survive in the desert and pre desert existence. Prey and predators would be smelt and heard in the day and at night. Touch is a reflection of the lower pain threshold the original man had necessary for survival. He had to be careful not to be injured or he and his family could well die. Heightened vision was necessary to spot prey and predators. Later in the tribe there would be many eyes to look out for things. The original man only had his own and his wife's eyes.

An interesting interaction occurs with the senses and the degree of focus that the original mind is capable of. I have observed an ability to ignore pain whilst this mind is focussed on a particular activity. I recall somebody trying to light a fire and being so focussed on this that they didn't notice they had burnt their own finger. Yet at the same time this person was so sensitive he didn't like new trousers because they felt uncomfortable.

<u>Clumsiness, balance difficulties, difficulty judging distances, height, depth, gross or fine motor coordination problems</u>: The original mind only ever killed at close quarters with a hand axe to the throat of the prey. The tribe developed hunting with spears and use of these tools meant improved coordination and spatial awareness were necessary for success. The basic techniques that are needed for hunting with spears are reflected in the way we throw balls today. There is accuracy and the ability to judge distance. The tribal mind developed these abilities through the process of natural selection. Those that developed the abilities survived. The original mind took a different course in evolution. It took the farming route, which is actually cleverer than running around throwing spears. This evolutionary course did not select for the ability to use the spear and the natural characteristics that evolved for that purpose. This is why a large hammer is the preferred tool for fine technical adjustments to delicate farm machinery.

<u>Difficulty in recognizing others faces</u>: There should be no natural understanding of faces in the original mind. The original man didn't originally live with other people hence

there was no need to remember which face belonged to which person. This ability developed in the tribe, as it was necessary to be able to tell who was who for the tribe to function efficiently.

Self-stimulatory behaviour to reduce anxiety, stress or to express pleasure: By accessing more basic body functions the original mind can override conscious thought. In the original man's time this would not have been necessary because the life style then would have meant the mind and body would have been occupied on a fairly constant basis or exhausted. In modern life physical exhaustion doesn't happen very often and it is hard to exhaust the mind. Some of this behaviour can appear a little odd; however in the original existence there was nobody to see it.

Self-injurious behaviour: This is simply a way to override conscious thought in the original mind when self-stimulatory behaviour isn't enough. Physical pain gives the mind a rest from other problems it is grappling with and provides relief. This type of injury may be kept private or it may be displayed as a cry for help and attention.

Nail-biting: I do this. It helps deal with boredom mainly.

Unusual gait, stance or posture: This is a lack of self-awareness and self-image. The original man had nobody to see him. The unusual style of walking that can be seen in some autistic people is how we used to walk. There can be a tendency to slouch, which served evolutionary purpose in the desert existence where we needed to look to the ground for food. In the tribe the animals we caught were much larger and the tribal mind evolved to look straight ahead. Posture also served a purpose of communication. By standing straight and tall you gave the message that you were somebody to be taken account of. The sloucher was somebody who wasn't to be taken account of and this was fed through into sexual behaviour. Women preferred the confident upright man.

Low apparent sexual interest: The underlying interest in sex in the original mind is likely to be the same as for the tribal mind as sex drive came from a common ancestor before the original man. This behaviour was substantively formed in the trees and was promiscuous. Food was abundant at this time and females didn't rely on males in the provision of food. Each could have as many partners as they wished and it didn't matter. When we came to life in the desert we found ourselves at the opposite extreme. This was a time of monogamy and limited sexual activity born out of stress. In the tribe things became different. The tribal existence was easier than the past original existence in the desert. Relationships became more intense in their passion. The need for monogamy was reduced and the short-lived love affair evolved. Children were cared for communally in the tribe and there wasn't the need for a couple to remain together for the whole duration needed to rear children. We see an increase in sexual activity stimulated by the existence of choice. No longer one partner for life - the good times were back. The original mind has the desire from programming in the trees but it's constrained by a natural thought of affordability. The original man could only afford to feed one woman and woman one man and this natural characteristic has been inherited by the original mind today.

Depression and Anxiety: Depression arises in the original mind through a lack of control. It needs to be in control to be satisfied. Unfortunately however control now often lies in other people's hands. This can lead to depression anxiety and stress. This can be particularly the case if you have to deal with some of the baboons in the public authorities these days. In personal relationships we can find two fairly uncompromising personalities impacting on each other. Neighbours can also impact on each other in a negative way. Ones man's obsession with his leaf blower in pursuit of the perfect garden is in conflict with his neighbour's pursuit of peace and tranquillity. Cooperation and compromise is all but essential in modern living.

Unfortunately the original mind is not naturally adapted for this and if it hasn't learnt the art of compromise it can have some problems.

Sleep difficulties: The original mind can become over stimulated. In the original family's time this would have proved useful when hungry. They would have kept going into the night to find food. Sleep difficulties were reported in Winston Churchill I believe. He slept for four hours a night. This gives some guide of the sleep necessary when the original mind is in a heightened state of arousal. In the original family's time it is unlikely that this peak state of arousal would have lasted for too long. The body would have become too weak from hunger to function properly if food wasn't found within a relatively short period of time. Obviously in modern times hunger isn't an issue and hence sleep difficulties can persist if the mind remains in a high state of arousal. This tends to occur more now than it did in the past due to a lack of physical activity and increased stimulation from modern living.

Difficulty expressing anger excessive or bottled up: Anger is likely to be a characteristic from early evolution. Many animal species display anger when threatened or are competing for food or sex. In the tribe anger had to be moderated to a greater extent than in the original single-family existence. In the tribe people had to live and function together. Punching each other's lights out did not serve to create social harmony. Equally however anger served a purpose of a warning in the tribe when one member's actions were out of order. The tribal mind evolved to moderate the effects of anger by using display rather than physical aggression. For the original mind there is no natural moderation as there is in the tribal mind, which leads to a wide variety of reaction to it just depending on learnt behaviour of self control.

Flat or monotone vocal expression: Language is fully learnt by the original mind. As such vocal expression is also fully learnt. The tribal mind naturally developed

160

language and with it natural vocal expession. The expression and words all formed part of a system of communication that was essential for the tribe to function. As language is fully learnt by the original mind its development can suffer if that mind is particularly obsessed with something else. I have noticed odd language particularly in a number of high achieving sports people that I get to hear on the television.

Difficulty with initiating or maintaining eye contact: This will be during conversation. The original mind has to access all conscious thought during conversation, as there is no natural understanding of language. It could perhaps be similar to lying in the tribal mind hence the tendency to look away while thinking. Eye contact evolved in the tribe so each member knew who was talking to whom. It is not natural to the original mind as there was no reason for it to develop in the original single-family existence.

Elevated voice volume during periods of stress and frustration: This is due to a lack of self-awareness and patience in the original mind. Mind you I would say all people can be prone to the odd rant so there is not much unusual in this.

Strong food preferences and aversions: This is linked to a more sensitive sense of smell hence taste and a more sensitive sense of touch hence appreciation of texture of food. Further more diet in the past was quite limited in its variety. In the trees we ate fruit and this is why children like sweet things. After this we ate mainly meat. There wasn't any broccoli or cabbage then for children to have to endure. The original mind can be particularly unwilling to try anything different due to its less compromising nature. The tribal mind is more compromising and less sensitive to taste and texture. This leads to a wider taste and this can be reflected in the quality and variety of cuisine in different countries. It is the reason why the French can eat garlic snails. I shudder at just the thought.

Bad or Unusual, personal hygiene: This can equally be scrupulously good personal hygiene. It's simply because the original mind doesn't have intuitive self awareness. It can either under compensate for this or over compensate depending on what's learnt. When combined with obsession we can see excess behaviour as in the repeated washing of hands to make sure they are clean.

A common feature of the autistic or original mind is the way in which it interprets words and sentences in a literal manner. This arises from this minds natural honesty and it assumes that other minds are equally honest and they say what they mean. The tribal mind however doesn't use language in this direct way. It evolved to use honesty in a beneficial way to itself and the tribe as a whole. For instance you ring the council and they say the person you want to talk to is in a meeting. This doesn't mean that this person is necessarily in a meeting its just they don't want to talk to you as it might involve them having to do some work. In order to avoid offence a white lie is used. The literal manner in the way the original mind naturally operates is actually used in Law. We interpret written statutes in a literal way in order to try and stick with a fixed point of reference. If we tried to interpret the intentions of the person behind the words then we venture into the world of speculation, which leads to all sorts of problems with variation of meaning.

Another characteristic that is frequently linked to Asperger's Syndrome is a lack of common sense. Common sense is defined as: native good judgement. It is natural ability as opposed to learnt ability. When you start to think about it though it becomes rather harder to define. What action makes sense? A decision can be logical based on a narrow view; however take a wider view it can become illogical. I think it is this that is being observed. For instance lets take the simple act of opening a door as an example. Now I am not sure anybody would be this stupid but you never know. Common sense would say that you press down the handle and push the door open. This is a logical decision taken on a narrow focused route. The door doesn't open. The door must be locked - another logical decision on a narrow focused route and so you go away. Taking a wider perspective the door could open by either pushing it or alternatively pulling it and in fact you needed to pull it open to go through. What we are seeing is decision-making following a narrow focussed track and failing to take in sufficient information to arrive at the logical conclusion. The term common refers to most, as in most people, and they did evolve to take a wider view than the original mind. When we take a wider view of Asperger's Syndrome for instance it doesn't make common sense. How can conclusions from National Socialist political science be taken seriously when it concerns people? We know there is nothing wrong with Jewish people or Gypsies so why should we think they were right about Asperger's Syndrome?

The model for evolution that I have presented fits the description of what is currently classified as a mental disability. To me this classification is wholly wrong. It is similar to the nineteenth century view that the black African was an inferior race which, was simply a judgement based on ignorance.

What Hans Asperger's work did although it is not yet realised is give us a critical step in human evolution, which so far has not been recognised. There has been a general belief that we are social creatures and it was social ability that made the human race what it is. There is a vision of all our ancestors hunting together in a tribal cooperative group. Now what if that general perception is not true. To me it does not fit how we behave today. The single family is the bedrock of human group behaviour and most people in the world live in this way. For me this means that the single family existed as a crucial stage in human evolution. Rather than sociability ensuring human survival I actually believe it was the exact opposite that was true. Anti social behaviour kept people spread out in the desert and it was that behaviour that allowed mankind to survive in a place

where other more cooperative hominoid species could not
live.

Chapter Eighteen

The evolution of the geography of the human world

The current geography of the human population of the world follows a pattern that is dictated by the two basic human personalities. This is significant especially in the area of world politics. For instance the recent Iraq fiasco should never have happened had there been an understanding of the geography of human behaviour. The pattern we can see is based on migration and can be best visualised in the form of a circle. We have the original place of origin in East Africa at the centre of the circle and the final migratory destinations at the edges of the circle. As far as behaviour is concerned we have a concentration of tribal minds at the centre and a concentration of original minds at the edge. This doesn't mean that we just have original minds at the edge there are plenty of tribal minds as well. It means that the greatest number of original minds is concentrated at the edge. An example would be Silicon Valley in California. In the body of the circle we have varying balances of the two with a tendency towards tribal behaviour nearer the centre and original behaviour towards the edge.

Evolutionary expansion of the human population took the form of migration driven from the centre in East Africa outwards. Hunting would again become the dominant behaviour when environmental conditions allowed, as the tribe needed it to maintain status. This activity was an integral part of tribal life and continued not because it was the only option available but because it was necessary for the tribe to function. The herds of herbivores would be the object for pursuit. We see a pattern of later migrants displacing the earlier ones with the earliest migrants of all eventually pressed out to the furthest edges of the world. DNA testing has established that the Australian aborigine is genetically the most distant from the modern African. This is because the aborigine was one of the first to leave Africa. It seems implausible that the aborigine would have chosen to walk all the way from Africa to Australia because he wanted to and he didn't. He was pushed out from land closer to the original centre bit by bit as later more competitive migrants arrived. He entered Australia at around 60,000 years ago.

The pattern of migration with waves of migrants being progressively displaced would have meant that humans increasingly adopted a more battle like mentality. The first people out of Africa were the least aggressive and the poorest fighters. The later ones to migrate would become more aggressive with the most violent holding the original central area. We see this pattern of behaviour today. Africa seems to enjoy more fighting on a regular basis than the rest of the world put together. Africans are naturally the most competitive people. Fighting is the way in which this competitiveness is expressed and is the reason why they held the original central territory. The tribal mind was however naturally limited in its fighting capability to small-scale skirmishes. Casualties on any significant scale would undermine confidence. Each man of the tribe had an inbuilt compassion for his fellow men and the feeling of grief when they were killed. This compassion would limit fighting in the early migrations with tribes spreading out rather than fight to hold land.

We are going to look at the migration into Europe as an example to see how cultures were formed. There is a pattern that can be seen based on the existence of the two personalities. This pattern varies from north to south and can also be distinguished in terms of specific locations where cultures would originally form. In the north we see barbarian cultures and in the south civilisation. Both are in fact remarkably similar and are only distinguished by circumstance. The difference arose out of war. In terms of the specific locations from where barbarian culture and civilisation arose this was formed out of competition between tribal and original minds for land. Original minds were pressed out through the pressure of competition with the tribes to the least favoured land.

Around 43,000-40,000 years ago the world experienced a particularly arid phase. This coincides with the arrival of the first Homo sapiens in Europe. Lack of food and the pressure of competition for the meagre resources in East Africa drove migration north. However there were people already living in the north but they weren't like us. These people had occupied Europe for a long time before and they were the Neanderthals. This would be significant because it would create a human culture and maybe even a psychology that survives to this day and that is the behaviour of the warrior.

Previous migrants had wisely avoided venturing into the European fortress home of the Neanderthals. This was partly due to the bad weather then but also out of fear. The Neanderthals were a frightening species. This fear went all the way back to the time when man was persecuted by relative hominoid gangs. The new migrants to Europe however had one amongst their number who wasn't afraid and this was their religious teacher the shaman. This man wasn't like the people around him as he had an original mind. He had become part of the tribe back in Africa when the original family had provided the tribe with food in the time of need. He had been ordained by God to venture into the Neanderthals lair and had the confidence of his belief. From the shamans confidence the tribe derived confidence. He was their guiding light and their protector.

The shaman as protector did not only limit himself to religious matters of the mind but also took an interest in the human body. He became doctor to the tribe and would concern himself with the sick. This relationship between mental and physical well being would be significant in establishing the shamans position in the tribe. The Christ was recognised as a religious figure and his ability at healing the sick was part of what gave him the credibility he had. He however was not unique in this ability for healing was part of the duties of a shaman and one of their powers.

Modern day doctors are descendents of this profession and they still need the characteristics that made the shaman successful. These characteristics are the ability to transcend tribal human emotion of grief when dealing with death. They also need the ability to transcend tribal compassion when performing surgery. It is only by seeing the body as an object rather than a person that the cut can be made. The shaman's ability as a doctor and as a religious leader would combine together to provide the most significant man in history.

The shaman was a completely indispensable man. He was the most important person in the tribe and would take over control in the time of strife to come as we advanced into Europe. This would create a structure of organisation that survives in companies today. The shaman was the director and the chief was the manager. The shaman knew which direction he wanted the tribe to take. The chief had the natural ability to organise the men to function as a single fighting group.

The northern wars

The earliest Homo sapien remains in Europe date from around 40,000 years ago. Neanderthals are thought to have died out around 30,000 years ago. This gives us the potential for a 10,000-year war. Over such a time period the conflict must have been fought on a fairly sporadic basis. As is likely territory would be taken in the south with the gradual push north as the human population expanded. The Neanderthals were physically better suited to living in the cold. Their bodies had adapted over a long period of time to the environment. For the Homo sapien it was a different matter. He was from distinctly warmer climes and found the north rather chilly. The Neanderthal should have held his ground in peaceful circumstances however these were not peaceful times.

It would be nice to think that the human race is a peace loving species that dwelt quietly alongside the Neanderthals in loving harmony. This would however be denying reality. People have fought wars on a regular basis throughout recorded history with pretty much one occurring at least every generation. We had the religious wars between Christians and Muslims through the crusades. There have been various wars between Catholics and Protestants. Today there is Islamic terrorism against the attempted expansion of the Western capitalist empire throughout the world. These wars are based on a belief that they should be fought in the name of God. The shaman had the same beliefs.

The shaman was a general in the wars against the Neanderthal people. The tribal chief was the captain and the one that would be involved in the actual fighting. The chief had compassion for the welfare of his men that the shaman hadn't got. The chief wanted to keep his men in the world of the living. The shaman wasn't too bothered which world the men found themselves in be it the living or the dead. The shaman was single minded and victory was his sole aim in the name of God.

The Neanderthal was by no means a wimp or inferior species in the environment of the north. The men were tough, strong and fearsome killers. These people would hunt woolly mammoths, which was by no means an activity for the faint hearted. The Neanderthal man was much stronger than the Homo sapien. He had a stocky body with short strong limbs. These characteristics gave these people better adaptation for hunting. They were less prone to limbs being broken when bringing down large game. The Homo sapien however had a characteristic that had split man from the other hominoid species from when they all lived in Africa in a past time. Men were faster runners than Neanderthals and it was running that made the difference.

Between the chief and the shaman battle tactics were established. The chief could not tolerate heavy casualties befalling his men. The shaman instilled the belief that fight they must in the name of God. The practical solution reached was the guerrilla war. Man would wage a war of hit and run. Head to head conflict was too dangerous. A Neanderthal could break a man's arms or legs with his bare hands. If caught there was no chance of survival in the hands of a Neanderthal man.

Tribal men had established natural throwing abilities with the improvement of spears. Killing big game at close quarters had always been a risky business for all hominoids. The stone tipped spear had been developed for throwing. Earlier purely wooden spears were designed for simply thrusting and just bounced off when thrown. The sharp stone tipped spears were a throwers tool and would now be a throwers weapon. The spear would be the mainstay of the Homo sapien arsenal in the Neanderthal wars and guerrilla warfare were the tactics used.

The shaman however was never a man to sit on his laurels and constantly wanted better progress. It was not in his genetic makeup to sit still. He still had the mental programming from the time of great austerity in the desert and this meant he would not stop. In the shaman's great wisdom he decided on an especially grim tactic of war to be used. It has to be born in mind that this man had no natural compassion for there had been no other people to be compassionate about other than the family in the original existence. The tactic that the shaman brought forth was that of genocide.

Genocide is abhorrent to us; however it has undeniably happened and even so in recent times. During the Second World War Hitler embarked on a program of genocide to eradicate the Jews. In recent years genocide has been committed in Rwanda. This behaviour is unfortunately part of human history and I believe the first act of genocide was against the Neanderthal people. There are no records of this murder and I believe this arose out of guilt. Even today there is a desire to cover them up and deny that they ever happened. This is especially the case for those that commit them. We committed genocide against the Neanderthal people and have covered it up. They didn't die out by chance.

Killing a fully-grown Neanderthal man was tricky at best. It was a case of getting close enough to throw the spear but with enough distance to allow for a quick get away if you missed. There was also a good chance that the kill would be by no means instant. A thrown spear lacks the penetration power of one that is held. However it was only the very brave or very stupid that would dare to get close enough to a Neanderthal to stab him.

A safer tactic by far was to kill the women and children and this is the tactic that would be increasingly adopted. Unfortunately for the shaman the tribe didn't quite have the same level of motivation as he did. They wanted to enjoy life and a war of genocide wasn't really the sort of entertainment they were looking for. The tribe liked the easy life. They liked dancing, recreation, having sex and generally enjoying themselves. The shaman struggled to motivate the tribe; they just did not share in his belief to the same extent. The shaman needed men that would share in his belief. The shaman needed men that could endure a hard life and weren't looking to enjoy themselves. He needed men that were not that interested in dancing and seduction. These men did exist and they were the shaman's own children and the children of other shamans.

There was an established practice of inheritance of the shaman's position by the eldest son when the shaman died. The eldest son would learn the shaman's knowledge from his father and become shaman when his time came. There were however the shaman's younger sons and although one or two may find a specialised position as craftsmen in the tribe there were ones that were surplus to requirements. These men lacked the social graces and understanding of the tribal mind. They did not fit in with the hunt and were not part of the team. They didn't have the natural sexual prowess that the men of the tribe had. Tribal women didn't find them attractive. These men had the same original mind as the shaman but were without position. It was natural in the tribal mind not to like difference and the original mind was different. These men would find themselves dispossessed and cast out. The sons of shamans became the unwanted

It would however not be just the sons of shamans that were the unwanted for the daughters of shamans were also not wanted. These women also lacked social ability. They could not naturally fit in with tribal ways. They were naturally monogamous and hadn't developed the sexuality that the tribal women had. They were not attractive as they were not fun. They could not dance seductively and didn't take the same pleasure in sex that the other women did. These women would be pushed out by the tribe and also become the unwanted. There was however somebody that did want these people and this was the shaman of the north. He had a war to wage in the name of God and he needed manpower.

The shaman's new tactic of genocide did have its down side. The Neanderthal men that had their women and children killed would not take it lying down and retaliation was inevitable. They now had nobody to provide and care for and so could devote their time to fighting the invaders that had inflicted the torment they now endured. It must be remembered however that mankind had been born out the same treatment and the natural fear he had of relative hominoid species had come from being persecuted in the same way. Mankind however now returned the persecution on an altogether different scale. This was industrialisation of the business of killing.

The wars intensified and Homo sapiens were increasingly forced to take up fortified protected positions from Neanderthal attack. These positions would be in caves on cliff faces. Ladders would be used to access the cave, which could be pulled up in times of trouble. These defensive positions were the predecessors to hill forts and castles that would be built for the same purposes in a future time although for protection against different enemies. With intensification of the war and retaliation by the Neanderthals battle tactics evolved. The front would now be pushed a long way from where the women and children lived. Bands of fighters would be sent off to fight on the front and these men would spend weeks if not months away from home. The wars would attract men with a certain mentality. This mentality was one of a psychopathic and generally intemperate disposition. The barbarian was born and it was to the north they went in the pursuit of war.

The shaman of the north may have been a psychopathic genocidal maniac however he would draw people to him. As illogical as it sounds this behaviour has happened in recent times and still happens today. Adolf Hitler managed to offer the German people purpose to their existence in his psychopathic policies of the Third Reich. The shaman likewise offered a place and purpose to the dispossessed. He created an army of out casts and a culture developed to make these people function as one. These people didn't have natural social abilities. They had neither natural empathy nor natural compassion for each other. They did not have the natural ability to function as a group and so in its place was created an artificial one. Culture would in time become more important than natural innate behaviour and it was all born out of a lack of natural ability.

The culture of the north was based on religion and war. By fighting the war men would find their way to heaven or Valhalla. All people fear death and this fear should in theory have prevented war. Belief however serves to

173

override the natural fear in order that a war can be fought. The belief in a warrior's heaven would become an integral part of the evolving cultures of the north and it would be this belief that would drive the Neanderthal wars to their conclusion. There was one crucial artificial concept that made all this work and that was honour.

A man's honour would become prized above all else even life itself. Honour was integrally intertwined with religion. A man could not pass into heaven or Valhalla without his honour intact. The code of honour needed for original minds to fight together would have been fairly simple. The main foundation of the code would be not to leave your comrades in the face of danger. The temptation to abscond would be the natural reaction however with the group divided defeat becomes more likely.

To counteract the temptation to run came the concept of shame in cowardice. This prevented the group splitting in the face of adversity. The men would stand and fight together. This basic cultural code would through time be artificially expanded to eventually give us the codes of honour of the knights of the middle ages and the gentlemen of the eighteenth and nineteenth centuries. These were cultural codes born out of this original warrior's code of honour.

The warrior gained a special status in the eyes of the human world. They were respected men. They were attractive to women. They were imbued with a mythical magic and this was in no small part due to the shaman. These men were his creation. They were his disciples placed on earth by the Almighty to do Gods will. These men were the ancestors of people who would come to be the barbarians of the north. Our culture has been deeply influence by these people and we have in part inherited their mental characteristics.

The Neanderthal wars bred cooperation between tribes. Whilst there was a common enemy mankind would function as one. Industry would develop in the south that would feed the front on the north. It is in times of war that humanity makes some of its most rapid advancements. The warriors would be paid homage as the original farmer was paid homage when the tribe had been starving in Africa. The shaman had descended from the farmer and likewise the warrior from the shaman. All these people were revered and were paid for the special contributions they made to humanity.

The Neanderthal people became extinct around thirty thousand years ago. The very last ones had been hunted to the edges of the world. The warrior people would form the groups that would become the Celts, Vikings, Saxons, Angles, Jutes and Huns and probably quite a few others in the north of Europe. These people were successful fighters in the wars; however their nature was less competitive than that of the tribe. When we think of Vikings for instance we find they were very successful warriors yet they came from the particularly unsought after area of freezing Scandinavia. The south of France is a much nicer place to live. We find that the locations that the great warrior cultures would emerge from would not be sought after prime areas but the undesirable peripheries. This all arose from pressure of competition with the tribes.

Once the Neanderthal wars were over the tribes would migrate into the newly conquered lands. Without a war to fight the original warriors dispersed to live in their natural single-family groups. Through pressure of competition these original families were gradually pressed out to the least favourable land. It is in these places that the descendants of the original warriors congregated together and from there we would see the emergence of the great warrior cultures. We will take a look at one of these cultures and I have chosen the Celts.

Contemporary Roman writers have described the Celts as living in tribes of 20,000 to 250,000 in number. The description of tribe however is not accurate. The natural size of a tribe is only a couple of dozen people plus children. Try and increase this size and natural cooperative behaviour is insufficient for the group to function. To live in large groups an artificial code of behaviour is needed and for the Celts that code was based the warrior's code of honour. Roman observations of the Celts described them as especially keen to engage in war. This enthusiasm was engrained in their culture for it was through war that honour was gained.

The word Celt has been translated from various roots. One translation is from an Indian-European word "quell" meaning elevated or noble. Another word from the same source is "Kel" meaning hidden. A derivative of this word in English is the word "kilt" a garment the Scottish wear to conceal their personal parts. These translations describe the natural behaviour of the original minds that formed the Celts. These people are believed to originate from around the source of the river Rhine in the Europe. They hid in the mountains away from the tribes and from there formed into the Celtic people. The kilt is a garment of modesty. Modesty again is the natural behaviour of the original mind and is the same sexual restriction that is portrayed in the Bible with Adam and Eve and the fig leaves.

Celtic culture was based on an artificial class system. At the bottom of the system is the working class. I suspect the tribes that the Celts subsumed in their expansion tended to find themselves generally in this class. The class up from this was the warrior class. Next up was the shaman's professional class and these were the Druids. These people performed all the functions that the shamans had performed in the past. They were religious leaders doctors and scholars. They were also now deciders on legal matters based on the law that had developed to provide structure to Celtic society.

At the top of Celtic society were kings and queens. It is quite interesting to note that women were imbued with a similar status to men. This is a characteristic from the original desert existence where there was no status. Our typical perception of the tribal chief is one of a man. We do not think of the chiefess and in fact there is no such word. We do find a natural difference in the status of men and women in the tribal world and this is reflected in the Muslim religion. There is also a contrast in the original world in so far as kings and queens were not religious leaders. Religion has natural foundation for men communing with God to see future. A woman has a man to look to for future. The status of king or queen needed no such natural difference and perhaps the most famous of all Celts was in fact a woman queen Boudica.

As the cultures of the north were developing the south was developing but in a slightly different fashion. Advances were made in tool making by the craftsmen of the tribes. Religion had evolved and the seeds were set for the creation of the classical civilisations.

The cause of civilisation

I will provide my definition of the term civilisation. "Civilisation is the artificial creation of rules of behaviour".

The question is why would we create artificial rules of behaviour? The answer lies in the type of people that came to live together. Artificial rules were set out in order that people who were not naturally able to cooperate were able to live and function together as a group in just the same way as the warriors had done.

The last cold period of our Ice age ended around 12,000 years ago. This date is significant as it marked the coming of a time of plenty with a more temperate environment. It would mean that the pressure on the human population that gave rise to migration would diminish and a period of stability set in.

It is the location of the classical civilisations that is of crucial interest. Be it Mesopotamia, The Yellow River in

China, Greece, Egypt or Rome they all have one thing in common. These places are in periphery locations. They are not the prime central areas of choice. In being periphery locations they were not subject to the competitive forces that the prime areas were subject to. Mesopotamia was started in the marshes of the river Euphrates and Tigris. Egypt is in desert at the edge of Africa. The Greek civilisation was very much located on the Greek islands and Rome was formed at the edge of a straggly peninsular called Italy. Tribes would on occasion fight each other for the prime areas where the large game roamed; however the peripheries would enjoy peace for generations in this time of plenty. Innovation would drive agriculture through drainage and irrigation to make these otherwise unsought after areas into survivable and eventually prosperous places.

Mesopotamia

The first known civilisation I have found is Mesopotamia, which is in modern day Iraq, that country we recently had the wisdom to invade for some reason. The name Mesopotamia is the ancient Greek name for land between two rivers. Civilisation in Mesopotamia is dated back to around 3500-4000BC and is recorded as just a little earlier than ancient Egypt. The location for this civilisation is significant and in particular the legend that describes the land. Mesopotamian legend said that the world was made out of a watery waste. Now this is not true for much of the earth however it was true of their world. The land of Mesopotamia was indeed marshland that the people drained to create farmland. Although this land was very fertile once drained it was not, at the time it was occupied, prime real estate at all.

The people that occupied the marshes at the ends of the Tigris and Euphrates rivers were not naturally cooperative people. They were descendants of the original single-family from Africa. They naturally lived a single-family lifestyle and were farmers. The tribes had pushed these people out from all the previous lands they had occupied. They finally found a refuge in the marshlands of Mesopotamia. In this place they found peace and in time prosperity. The tribes did not come into the marshes because there was no big game there for them. The single family could survive on much scarcer resources just as it had in the desert in Africa. The marsh provided food in the form of fish, birds and eggs. Above all the marsh was safe and this gave the opportunity to invest and acquire capital in the form of livestock. As livestock was acquired so marshland was drained to create grazing land. It was by coincidence I believe that this land with its alluvial deposits made extremely good arable land.

Records of the origins of cereals seem to suggest they have come from the Middle East. On the evidence it looks probable that arable farming started with the first classical civilisations. This type of farming would need to have coincided with the rebirth of the concept of personal land ownership. Livestock can be grazed on common land; however arable crops need a field to grow them in. There needs to be a concept of land ownership for without it anybody could harvest the crop. This concept is natural to the original mind.

In Mesopotamia the original minds that lived in the marshes carved out their own fields from those marshes using ditches. These ditches formed boundaries, which drained the land, kept livestock in and showed where each man's land was. The true farm was born and ownership of the land was beyond dispute for the farmer had created that land with his own hands. Later written evidence on a clay tablet from around 1300BC records a map of land ownership near the city of Nippur showing canal or ditch boundaries along with the name of the owner or occupier of each plot of land.

The people of Mesopotamia were naturally capitalists and as such expansion of land and livestock would be their natural behaviour. With expansion comes a surplus of supply over that needed for simple self-sufficiency. With excess food tends to come excess children. Some of these people would further extend farmland however there is always a limit to land and even bog availability and so some would need to find other occupations. The children of the farmers just as before in Africa and beyond became shamen and craftsmen. This time however rather than being supported by the tribe they were paid by the farmers for their services.

Now if you have any experience of trying to get original minds to naturally cooperate, as I have, you will know that this is not easy. They do not have the naturally cooperative nature of the tribal mind and each wants everything their own way. Compromise is not a naturally occurring function as it is by necessity in the tribal mind. In the original single-family existence there was nobody to compromise with apart from the wife and that was hard enough. Into this void of a natural ability to get along with each other would come innovation in the form of artificial codes of behaviour. This was the creation of civilisation.

The first forms of cooperative behaviour between original minds would be through trade. Now there existed farmers, shamans, craftsmen and trade existed between these people each buying services from the other. It would be the shaman who would move development forward to create the things we recognise as classical civilisation. The substantial stone structures that we know of are religious in nature. Had the farmer been responsible for the development we would have had giant grain stores. Had the craftsman been responsible we would have had a DIY store.

The Shaman

The shaman was responsible for communicating with God and interpreting God's will. This was not a free service people had to pay for it with the food and goods they produced. Payment had to be made if the goodwill of God was to be secured. This goodwill took the form of favourable climatic conditions. A good year for the harvest and God's favour had obviously been secured. A bad year for the harvest and obviously God's good will had not been secured. Now in the bad years you might suspect that the shaman could come in for some criticism. However he was an opportunist and could turn disaster into victory. A bad year could mean he had not found God's favour or it could mean he hadn't found the right Gods favour. There was the need for more Gods one for each risk. This sounds like insurance and that is exactly what it was although there was no payout if things went wrong just larger payments at renewal. This would lead to a plethora of Gods one for each problem the people faced and payment ensured the Gods goodwill. The shaman collected the payments and ended up with rather a lot of goats.

The cleverest shamans started to become wealthy individuals. This wealth was particularly in the form of livestock as this was the first form of capital. The shaman would need land to house his wealth. He could afford to pay people to drain or irrigate some land for him; however he could vastly increase his wealth by purchasing it. The very fact that the land of Mesopotamia was at risk of flooding would give him this opportunity. On occasion the floods would catch some farmers out. They didn't manage to harvest their crops or get their livestock to high ground in time. The livestock and crops would be lost to the floods and some farmers as well.

The farmers that survived but lost their livestock or crops had a problem. They still owned their land; however they had no food or capital to buy food. Into this problem stepped the shaman. The clever shaman was able to predict the flood and had moved his livestock to high ground in time. He had capital and wanted land. The unfortunate farmer that had been caught out had land but no livestock. He had no way of feeding himself and his family. The shaman would buy the land from these farmers with his stock and keep the farmer as his tenant with the farmer paying rent in the form of produce. The shaman became a landlord and overlord.

The shaman was a landlord, banker and accountant. He had power over the lives of his tenants. As the population grew and the fertile land was a finite resource his power increased. Competition between farmers grew as the number of people who wanted to farm grew with the expanding population. Unemployment started to become a problem. There were only so many jobs available. This economic environment gave the shaman great power through his wealth. He had tenants competing for his land and people looking to him for work.

The shaman could indulge his wealth and power in his main interest and that was his religion. He had resources available in terms of manpower and food. He could afford to pay his people to build a temple to the Gods and so this is what he did. One such temple is at a place called Uruk in Mesopotamia and dates from 3500 BC. It is estimated to have taken around 7500 man-years to build. The design of temples as ziggurat structures in Mesopotamia is an interesting link back in evolution. The people of Mesopotamia believed that the Gods lived in high places. They also believed they themselves originated in the mountains. This is a link that can be traced back in evolution to when we were pressed out to live in the mountains of East Africa.

Writing is an important part of classical civilisation and forms an artificial boundary between what we term history and prehistoric. For me the most interesting thing about writing as with all things is the reason for it in the first place. As with everything I believe there is a simple cause. There was the need for a fixed record of agreement between people. In other words there was the need for a contract. In Mesopotamia these agreements took the form of clay tablets, recording fields and crops with an example dating from 2800 BC. The clay tablet is likely to be a lease. The tablet shows the land let and the rent to be paid in the amount of crops to be given to the landlord. The farmer would pay his rent in arrears when he had produced livestock or crops to sell.

With an increasingly complex society cooperation between people increased. These people were not naturally able to function in a group and into this void would come law. Law is the creation of artificial rules of behaviour by which people's actions are governed. With the creation of artificial rules comes the need for everybody to know exactly what those rules are. This requires the rules to be set down literally in stone so that there is a fixed reference for people to go to.

There is an age-old problem with verbal communication and that problem is distortion of the message as it is passed from one person to the next. Each time a message is transmitted it changes slightly or sometimes not so slightly. After it has passed though several people the message is somewhat or even completely different to the original one that went out. This creates doubt in the spoken word and for original minds to function together there needs to be certainty as to exactly what the rules of cooperative behaviour are. Classical civilisation gave us the innovation of statute law. An example of this written law can be seen in the Louvre in Paris. Dating from 1790 BC this pillar or stele is black and taller than a man. On it Hammurabi I of Babylon sets out his laws in writing in order they are fixed and can be referred to by everybody. This was as long as they could read.

The classical civilisations are recognised with such reverence and respect because of the innovation they brought about. This innovation was born out of the minds that formed these societies. They were not constrained like the tribal mind with the concept that something could not be done. From this we see the like of things not seen in such quantity and quality before. Classical architecture and literature remains outstanding to this day.

The fall of classical civilisations and migration

Classical civilisations are particularly recognised for the urban living that they brought about. This form of living was created by original minds; however they are naturally the least likely to like it. The tribal mind with its naturally sociable nature is much better adapted to the urban environment where people are forced to be close together. Furthermore original minds are not naturally tolerant of autocratic rule. Each likes to have its own way. In the case of autocratic rule one mind gets a bit too much of its own way to the detriment of the others. Whilst the tribe may tolerate this, the original mind doesn't and either moves on or causes a revolution.

The classical civilisations would as they developed increase urbanisation and progress to autocratic rule with pharaohs and emperors. The result is a gradual migration of original minds away from these urban centres with tribal minds taking their place. This pattern of migration would continue through out history to the modern day and would have significant repercussions for the structure of the world. We see a picture of stagnation or decline in the old centres as the innovative original minds move out. New centres are created based on trade and industry and they themselves then stagnate or decline as they became congested and the original minds move on again. Places like Egypt, Mesopotamia, Rome and Greece would be left behind with other locations becoming the new innovative centres. One of perhaps the most unusual of these new places is Venice in Italy. The location of this city is on some of the least desirable land of all and is virtually built in the sea. Again we see an example of original minds being pressed out to the edge away from congestion and restriction. In Venice they created one of the major commercial centres of the middle ages.

Following the fall of the Roman military empire the warrior cultures would be the dominant forces of the dark ages.

184

Classical values were replaced with warrior values. We term this period the dark ages because unlike the classical period writing was not an integral part of the warrior existence. We therefore have comparatively few written records of this period in history. Prior to Roman occupation Britain had been a refuge to various migrants and after the Romans left would become home to more refugees.

In Britain we look back on empire and think how great we were. However it isn't the most competitive people that create greatness but rather the most innovative. Britain, like the location of the ancient Greek civilisation and that of Rome was on the edge of Europe. In the same way as people were pressed out to the locations of those civilisations people were pressed out to Britain. This island was not a prized central area. It was a refuge for the displaced. The people that sought refuge were the same as they always had been. These people were original minds pressed out by competition from the more central areas of Europe to the edges. They were Jutes and Angles from the peninsular that now forms Denmark along with Saxons from the Northern coast of Germany. On the West side of these people were the Franks and we know what the French are like. On the East were the Vandals a fairly nasty bunch of thugs. The Angles Jutes and Saxons were in something of a sandwich and it was their lack of competitiveness that pressed them out to Britain following the exit of the Romans.

As with the migrations to the locations of the first civilisations, migration to Britain would concentrate the innovative nature of original minds. The character of the British people is one of mild eccentricity. This character is born out of a lack of self-awareness and a lack of shame in being seen to do things differently. Eccentricity takes the form of behaviour and appearance with a wide range from no appreciation to an obsessive appreciation dependant on what is learnt. This character is fundamental to innovation and the reason for it. Innovators can only do things differently because they are not embarrassed by what people think of them. It was this character that marked Britain out from the rest of the world through innovation in the form of the industrial revolution. Out of this grew empire with Britain being the most powerful country in the world for a while. The behaviour of the people that drove the industrial revolution was typical of how the original innovative mind functions. Isambard Brunel was one such man. He was a migrant to Britain having come from France. He had all the obsessive qualities of the original mind. He had no concept of couldn't be done, created huge ships in iron and worked obsessively to death.

In Britain we see the cause for further migration of original minds to form the new world in America. British rule was made up of original minds competing against each other for control and balance. The Magna Charta was an important historical step in the start of democracy. This early form of democracy was to remove absolute power from the king. It was quite nicely stitched up in the favour of the other original minds however as only landowners and town burgesses were represented in parliament. The mass population did not have much of a say.

James I is a king that I find particularly worth mentioning when looking at the causes of migration. This king sought to reaffirm autocratic rule through fundamental belief. James I was a theorist and his theory was known as the divine right of kings. God was the ruler of the world, the king ruled on behalf of God. Therefore a monarch could not be disobeyed, just as God could not be disobeyed. Not every original mind however shared James I view. This is typical of original minds and a society with a large number of them has to be fairly tolerant. Britain at this time however wasn't quite the tolerant place it needed to be. One particular group that found themselves at odds with the king's view of how things should be were the Puritans. It was the environment created by James I that lead to Puritans moving to America and the formation of the USA.

Their values would become deeply engrained in American values.

The United States of America would become a refuge for original minds. This country reflects original values very clearly and the constitution is based on them. All people are created equal which is a commitment to original values with tribal status disregarded. It is the concentration of the innovative nature of its people that makes the United States the richest country in the world. The underlying belief that anything can be done is from the original mind. The American work ethic is one of long working hours and dedication. This is born out of long working hours and obsession from the original existence.

American sport is peculiar and rather unique to that country. They aren't as interested as other countries are in football or soccer as it is known there. This has arisen out of the original minds lack of competitiveness. Competition with other people evolved in the tribe. The original mind survived through innovation. Americans can sometimes seem brash or they are sometimes excessively polite and nice. This all stems from a natural lack of understanding of tribal manners, which in turn leads to a wide variety and reactions to offence. America is the home of the psychologist. This arises out of the naturally less stable nature of the original mind which leads to all sorts of odd behaviours, many driven by the natural obsessive tendencies. America created the nuclear bomb, which is the ultimate expression of the desire to avoid fighting. In the original existence we evolved to avoid killing each other.

The structure of the human world is explained by the current distribution of the different mind types and ties in generally with the state of a nation's development. We have the innovative original minds located in the most developed countries and at the other extreme tribal minds in the least developed. There are few original minds left in East Africa as most have now migrated away, which leaves a society with little ability to innovate or create wealth. Africa as things stand is destined for poverty unless original minds return, which is certainly a possibility for the future. At the other extreme are the countries that are the final destination for migration. These countries are the USA and Australia. Here we have the strongest concentration of original minds. This is quite interestingly illustrated by America and Australia's opposition to the Kyoto agreement to limit climate change. The original mind does not naturally have a social conscience, as there was nobody to be conscious of in the original existence. This behaviour is reflected in the policy of government of those countries. They do however have a point in the fact that likely future developing polluters are excluded from the agreement, which is a bit daft.

In terms of practical application of this behavioural structure for the world we need to consider the likely balance of behaviour for a particular country or region. For instance in the case of Iraq we might suspect that tribal behaviour would be the dominant force in view of its location. This means that the application of original values in the form of democracy and the rule of law may well not work. A tribal country looks to status for rule and it is not unnatural for such countries to adopt a firmer level of control. Naturally cooperative people are much better able to form themselves into groups of rebellion and as such require a stronger form of order to prevent anarchy. In places where the original mind is more dominant rebellions are much more unlikely. Getting two original minds to agree is difficult enough let alone several hundred. In these places better consideration is required for the individual rights of people if contentment with government is to be maintained. Should this contentment not be maintained then that government is going to find itself voted out of office. The balance of behaviour has to be considered if costly mistakes are to be avoided and we've made a few of those recently.

Human migration still continues with a flow of people out of the poorer tribal centres into the more affluent original peripheries. We do however see a shift in the types of mind that are moving now as Britain evolves into one of the old centres of civilisation. In the past it was a flow of original minds now we have the flow of tribal minds looking for work. This flow as in the past is into the urbanised centres. The Daily Telegraph recorded this pattern in an article dated 10th February 2005. The think tank Migrationwatch provided the change in Britain over the last ten years with 606,000 more people leaving London than arriving from elsewhere in the country. Over this period 726,000 people moved in to the capital from overseas. This change is referred to in America as the "white flight" and is a natural flow that has happened through history. I have to point out that this is not an issue of black or white in the conventional sense. Much of the immigration will be from white Eastern Europe. It is an issue of the two human personalities.

Chapter Seventeen

The evolution and psychology of religion

When we consider all aspects of human behaviour in the light of the existence of two personalities we can make sense of our religions. Prior to the Twentieth Century with the rise of science and psychology religion is where our personalities found refuge. In many respects it provides a much better form of guidance, reason and social coherence than blind belief in science can ever really offer. Just as we have evolved so religion has evolved through time and we will take a look at that evolution.

The first religion was one man with one God and this happened in the desert in the single family. We do however see our previous evolutionary experience influence our beliefs because they remain an integral part of us. To see the earliest recorded forms of religion we need to take a look at the earliest human records and these take the form of cave paintings.

Nicholas Humphrey from the Centre for Philosophy of Natural and Social Science at the London School of Economics compared cave art with drawings made by an autistic child. He set out his observations in "Cave art, autism and the evolution of the human mind 1998". Humphrey's makes the observation that he felt that the cave artists might have been operating at a pre-linguistic non-conceptual level. He says *"The makers of these works of art may actually have had distinctly pre-modern minds, have been little given to symbolic thought, have had no great interest in communication and have been essentially self-taught and untrained. Cave art, so far from being the sign of a new order of mentality, may perhaps be thought the swan-song of old."*

Nicholas Humphrey is basically right although he seems to portray the original mind in a slightly negative light. This mind is older than the tribal mind but to call it pre-modern is wrong. This mind created modern through the industrial revolution. A more accurate description would be pre-tribal. Our common perception in fact is that the tribal mind is the more primitive. Neither perception is true. The two together make modern man.

Michael Winkelman produced an article for the Cambridge Archaeological Journal 12 91-3,2002 titled "Shamanism and cognitive evolution". In his article he says, "cave art images represent shamanic activities and altered states of consciousness, and the subterranean rock art sites were used for shamanic vision questing".

Both these views tie in with our evolutionary account. The shamans did have original or autistic personalities. The artistic work they created was based on observation of what was seen rather than imagination based on what was told. They weren't interested in stories they were interested in fact. The shaman drew the animals of the day as he saw them. The animals he painted were worshiped because they were food and in essence the givers of life. He did also paint some of the predators of the day as representations of death.

The location of the art is significant in so far as the sites have religious significance. This significance arises from previous evolution and is a return to a place of origin. This place is the rock crevice although we had grown a bit since those times and so now it is the cave. Some of the rock art is located in the depths of the caves.

The significance of the location of art in the depths of the cave also comes from evolution. It is in these depths that our previous life is recreated and perhaps in some way remembered. This location is one of both protection and in essence life or birth but also a place of death. These two concepts arise out our ancient life in the rock crevice. At one time the depths of the crevice were a place of safety and life. Later in evolution the depths of the crevice were a trap and a place of fear and death. These two concepts from two periods in evolution combine in our emotions to provide a location that is deeply significant to the human mind. The cave naturally enhances religious worship of the cycle of life and death. Even today we still have the desire to return to the crevice and this is reflected in the desire to be buried. Cremation appeals to the natural desire to rise up to the heavens in smoke, which originates from the time we rose to the heavens in Pterosaur beaks. We don't see any desire to be recycled by being put in dog food because there is no natural origin to this even though it would perhaps be environmentally friendly.

What is the purpose of art? I think it would be fair to say that visual representation helps enhance the presentation of religious concepts. The location of the art suggests religious worship. However I think the art is a little more significant than that and this comes down to the manipulation of religion. Religion continually changed as it was passed down through the generations of shamans by word of mouth. Sometimes this was for better although knowing what the shaman was like more likely for worse and was inevitably going to be more expensive. The manipulation of religion was recognised as far back in time as 40,000 years ago in Australia. The Australian aborigines still use and reproduce religious imagery that was first set down all that time ago. In a future time religion would be set down in writing in an attempt to stop manipulation and provide a fixed reference. This is the purpose of the Bible and the other religious texts and people are extremely protective of their texts for the very same reason and that is to prevent manipulation.

It is however the manipulation of religion that leads to where we are today. We see a pattern of religion evolving to a point where it becomes too expensive and then a return occurs to the simple original worship. This pattern has been repeated throughout history and arises out of the capitalist personality of the original mind. Equally the return to the simple original worship comes from the original mind the only difference being who is paying and who is collecting the payment. Excess cost in religion is the very reason we have the most defining monuments in the earliest classical civilisations. It is also the reason we have the religions of today. So we will take a look at the process that gives us some of our greatest achievements.

In the classical civilisations the shaman would appeal to the human psychology in the religious structures he created. These were physical manifestations of the place that saw the birth of humanity in the form that we recognise as ourselves. They constructed mountains out of stone in the form of ziggurats and pyramids. By returning to the mountains so humanity returned to the place it was created and so to God the creator. The philosophy at the time may have been a little misguided but then that has happened throughout human evolution and still happens now. If you haven't got a mountain build your own and this is what the Mesopotamians and Egyptians did. This still happens in Las Vegas.

In Egypt we see the original mind take belief to the ultimate excess. The shaman's descendents the pharaohs would be thought of as living Gods. As Egypt's power developed it would begin to impact in a negative way on the people surrounding this great civilisation. The need for manpower increased as larger building projects were undertaken. The obsessions that the pharaohs had with their religion made it become too expensive. The people surrounding Egypt would come to pay the price for this extravagance. They were increasingly being enslaved to provide more workers to ensure that the monumental building works could be kept on schedule. This created resentment towards the numerous Gods and the power of the pharaohs and would bring forward the desire for a more economical religion.

193

The original religion was reborn and it came from the original single-family existence with a single God. The rules of behaviour that ensured the survival of the single-family at the time of great austerity in the desert were reaffirmed. These were written down in the form of the Ten Commandments and were set in stone so that they should never be forgotten again.

The Ten Commandments included the original behavioural rules along with a few more to stamp out the problems that had manifested themselves from the costs incurred by having lots of Gods. This basic simple and affordable religion in its various guises would be the one that would move forward and push out the old religions, which had become substantially corrupted. The desire for the reestablishment of honesty, which was the natural state for the original mind, would come via prophets preaching these original values. These prophets would be in time recorded in the Old Testament and the other religious works of the period.

The initial audience naturally had a desire for the values set out in the preaching's of the word of God. These people had original minds and lived the original lifestyle as shepherds. They were naturally men of capital and would never lose this behaviour because it was innate in their minds. They would in time become moneylenders to the world. These people were the Israelites and their cultural behaviour originated from the original single-family existence from which all humanity was born. Their beliefs would evolve into the Jewish religion and from this we would see a further split born out of the excesses at the time of the Roman Empire.

The coming of the Christ

The original religion, which had become the Jewish religion had like everything else developed so that status and wealth had become important. There was a desire for solace away from these costly values into which stepped

Jesus Christ. He represented a return to the original values again. These values were to discard status a concept from the tribe and taken to extremes by the Romans. Jesus taught the message of equality in the eyes of God. He promoted the abandonment of worldly possessions in favour of the pursuit of glory in heaven.

The messages sent by God through the Christ were in effect a reworking of the age-old balance between life and the concept of afterlife. In Egyptian world life was geared too strongly towards the afterlife with too much effort devoted to the pharaohs tombs. In the world at the time of the Christ the balance had shifted too far the other way. Worship to the Gods in the Roman world was for securing favour and help with living pursuits. These pursuits tended to generally involve killing people and extending areas of conquest. It was the concept of what the "Gods could do for man" that was the philosophy of the age. It is the concept of what "man could do for God" that was the message that Jesus wished to get across to the world.

Jesus Christ took values right back to the point in evolution of the single family in the desert. These values are the basis of the Ten Commandments. Jesus now promoted a conciliatory approach to these rules, which I believe arose out of the excesses of Jewish enforcement at the time. This excess behaviour is typical of unconstrained original minds. For instance the stoning of adulterers was a little harsh for having a bit on the side particularly bearing in mind that you're not supposed to kill. There was the promotion of forgiving trespass as expressed in the Lord's Prayer. Trespass in the original life in the desert was basically stealing. The punishments were excessively harsh with crucifixion as one of the consequences to look forward to. Jesus sought to moderate these excessive punishments through belief. He promoted the forgiveness of enemies not the killing of them. It was by not killing each other in the desert that man survived. He created a form of socialism with the concept of giving to the poor to counterbalance unrestrained capitalism both by Romans and Jewish.

The New Testament, just the same as had previously happened, mixed concepts from different times in evolution. These concepts were real and practically based. For instance Jesus fed the five thousand out of a few loaves of bread. This in itself is a mixing of the concept of the original-farmer in Africa feeding the tribe in its time of need along with the concept of feeding the religious soul. The healing that Jesus did was a mixing of the practical work of the shaman as a doctor with mental healing and well being derived from religious worship. The forgiveness of enemies was derived from the original existence when people evolved by not killing each other. The personal sacrifice that Jesus made for his people reflected the sacrifice made by the tribe in its cooperation with the original farmer for food. Every concept comes from evolution and has a natural place in the human mind. Jesus and the other prophets reaffirmed these natural concepts at a time when they were being forgotten. Above all the Christ gave something that was missing in us. That was compassion. This is not a natural feature of the original mind but is one God provided.

Christianity was taken up by the Roman Empire, which became the Holy Roman Empire following the collapse of its military based power. Early Christianity was an economical religion when it started out. Saints would travel through the country preaching their sermons and small churches were built. However the fact that it was taken up by the Romans who had already evolved expensive tastes meant as soon as the opportunity arose religion was going to cost a lot once more. The Catholic Church evolved to cater for the values of the tribal mind, which were the people Jesus sought to protect in the form of the mass population. The virgin was represented in the religion. The significance of the virgin girl comes from the tribe's sacrifice of the virgin girl to the farmer for food. The Catholic Church buildings were ornately and colourfully decorated. It was in the tribe that adornment and colour were used to signify status and sexual appeal. Catholics have confession because of the greater potential for temptation for departure from original values. The tribal mind is naturally more sexually competitive, which is seen as sinning by religion. The Catholic Church needs a strong authority to maintain religious discipline. It uses the fear of God in its fight against sin and has a strong opposition to divorce. This firm line works with tribal minds; however it a little less successful with original minds. They on occasion want to do their own thing, which doesn't quite fit in with Catholic authority.

The puritanical form of religion was born out the protestant movement formed by Martin Luther in the time of Henry VIII. This puritanical form of Christianity much better reflects the natural values of the original mind. The costs of the Catholic religion had increased with the magnificent cathedrals and churches that were built in the Middle Ages. Rather than money being spent on the welfare of the people we see the welfare of the church becoming rather more important. In just the same way as the Jewish religion had been born out of the cost of the Egyptian empire and Christianity out of the cost of the Roman Empire the same happened again. The puritans split from the Catholic Church and returned back to the basic values of the original mind.

The Quaker religion provides a clear view of how original values were reflected in the protestant faith. George Fox founded Quakerism in 1624. His mother's family were protestants who had suffered under the Catholics in the reign of Queen Mary. They were known to be a strong willed family who were independent in mind and spirit. George was taught to read. He was also taught to write and an unusual expression is used in describing the extent of this skill. He was taught to write as much as would serve to signify his meaning to others. In other words to use plain language. This is the natural state of the original mind's use of language. Because all ability is learnt there can be a plainness in it. This mind says what it means. George took a keen interest in sheep as a trader in livestock. A description of this interest at the time was " *he took most delight in sheep, so he was very skillful in them, an employment that very well suited his mind in several respects*". This links back to the original existence in the time of the tribe living as a farmer with the flock.

The basics of the Quaker belief are that God dwells within all men and women. This is an inward looking faith rather than an outward looking one. They do not look to religious leaders for guidance but rather to God within themselves. This links back to the original existence in the desert. The original man had only himself and God to look to. There were no other men to take guidance from. The Quakers believed that in the eyes of God all men were created equal. This links back to there being no status in the original existance. Status evolved in the tribe. Honesty was one of their guiding principles. They believed that people should always be honest so much so that they refused to swear they would tell the truth in front of a court. Their view was that they should always be honest and felt that by swearing to tell the truth implied they might not tell the truth in other circumstances. This comes from the original existence when there was only honesty.

The Quakers were pretty deterimind in their defiance of state rule. They refused to pay tithes to the Church of England and swear allegance to the King. They suffered for this defiance by having their assets confiscated and often found themselves in prison. Their personalities managed to endure this hardship because they were created in a time of suffering in the desert. We should have given up and died then but we did not. Our obsession made sure that we survived.

Pacifism is one of the Quaker principles. George Fox told the army when he was in prison in 1651 that he *"lived in the virtue of that life and power that took away the occassions of all wars."* This links back to the time in the desert. People evolved to keep out of each others way rather than to fight one and other.

The prohibition on consumption of alchohol is something that used to feature in some puritanical faiths. The reason why drinking is prohibited by religions geared towards the original mind is that it can become an addiction. The original mind tends to be more unstable than the tribal mind. It was formed in the hardest of times and still functions as if it lives in those times. The desire to escape this existence combined with obsession finds itself expressed by the consumption of alcohol, tobacco and various less legal substances. Prohibition serves to prevent the risk of problems arrising out of the addiction. Unfortunately prohibition also serves to make such religions rather unpopular with most original minds as they like the occassional beverage or three. There is an interesting contrast with the Muslim faith which also has a prohibition on the consumption of alcohol. This prohibition doesn't seem to affect the numbers worshipping the faith. The reason is that the mind type attracted to Muslim faith isn't that bothered about drinking anyway and so it doesn't put people off.

The Quakers humour can sometimes seem very odd as I found when I visited a factory that was heavily influenced by Quakerism. This humour was not really humour at all and involved a voice in the children's entertainment section that kept repeating, "let's have a right laugh". All very strange! This characteristic only existed intuitively in the tribal mind. Humour served the purpose of giving messages without causing offence. The original mind can learn humour and combined with obsession it can become the most popular humour of all. Equally it can be the worst humour of all.

The Quakers were entrepreneurs. They believed that because of restrictions placed on non-conformists in Britain from holding office or going to university they should place their energies into business. The Quakers had a large part in the industrial revolution although they don't sing about it because they are not interested in status. Birmingham in England is a place where Quakers congregated for this purpose. The factory I visited illustrated the natural dislike for the crowding that urbanisation creates. The Quakers that built the factory also built housing for its workers in a style that gave space and a feeling of a rural ideal.

It is through the industrial revolution that we come to the state of religion today. Darwin's "Origin of Species" may have been the catalyst for turning away from religion however we had started to worship science already. It had given us things that God had never before provided. Everybody could enjoy wealth, which had previously been the preserve of the few. Today it is the new religion and the scientist is the prophet of the modern world. Is he always right however? It would seem that in matters of the mind the answer to this is maybe not.

Chapter Nineteen

Evolution of working behaviour

The different mind types will tend to be drawn to different areas of work on the whole. The key things to consider are the basic natural characteristics of the two minds. For the tribal personality there is sociability that is of key importance. Work needs to be of a sociable nature to provide satisfaction and comfort. This arises out of the sociable nature of tribal existence. For the original mind there is the need for personal responsibility and control over the work that this mind carries out. This arises out of the original existence where there was only the original man and the wife to rely on and it was their personal decisions that meant success or failure. This all tends to lead to different areas of work and positions within the working environment suiting different mind types. The tribal mind is naturally suited to being told what to do. The original mind is naturally suited to doing the telling rather than the being told to. This tends to mean that higher positions suit original minds with middle and lower positions suiting tribal minds. The directors decide on direction and feed their ideas down to the managers who have natural ability at organising the workforce to carry out those ideas. That's how it should be anyway.

I now want to follow the evolutionary path of how work originated. This concept was established by the original mind and as such it is the original mind that is best suited to it. The tribal mind was the hunter and it is only in relatively recent times that the tribe has adopted work that original minds pioneered. This started with the adoption of farming to replace hunting in the late Stone Age. Following from this the tribal mind has found itself fitting in with work patterns established by the original mind. We will follow the evolutionary model of how work originated.

Farming is the first area of work that the original mind established and this first work still exists today. Farmers demonstrate classic signs of the original mind. They tend to work all the time when they don't actually have to. Clearly not all farmers have original minds but it's fairly easy to spot the ones that have. They can be awkward to deal with unless you understand them. They like to do things their own way and not be told what to do. They are often difficult to talk to. It's the way the original man was because he didn't talk in the original way of life. Farming now is not a sociable activity and is very much single family based. Related to farming is work with animals. Veterinary surgeons have compassion with animals and perhaps not with people particularly when it comes to their bills although mine is very good - he knows just how much large bills upset me.

I will leave the first true profession in evolution, which you may or may not have worked out and move onto the shaman. Today this is the vicar or religious leader. This profession should suit men who have passed the mid-life crisis and as such are in a position to commune with God. It was the passing of the point of natural death in the original existence that meant man could commune with God whilst he was still alive. Whether God chooses to commune with religious leaders is purely his prerogative which cannot be taken for granted. He chooses who he wishes to talk to regardless of status.

The shaman's role as religious leader also made him into another professional that we recognise today. This profession is closely related to the original communication of religious ideas and that is the profession of entertainment. Entertainment was an important way of making the tribe interested and understand religious teachings.

Today original minds dominate creative entertainment, even though the original mind is quite shy by nature. If this shyness is overcome by learnt behaviour and the introvert becomes the extrovert entertainment offers great potential. The tribal mind will find it hard to compete. It will be copying work that has gone before and that tends to lead to staleness. I'm sure we all know a few programs on the telly where that's occurred. The best comedy is actually a reflection of the original mind and it's relationships with other people. One program from the eighties that particularly springs to mind features a family of what are in effect wallies. It is the attributes of the original mind that are exceptional, interesting and funny at the same time that provides the entertainment. Early comedy through the likes of Charlie Chaplin was all based on observational humour, as there was no sound in early film. This is perhaps unintentionally a reflection of the evolution of comedy. It was animal behaviour observed by the original mind combined with tribal language and jokes that created modern situation comedy.

Music and singing is an area where the original mind dominates. This has been the case since Mozart. Modern pop is littered with original minds and it's that which makes it popular. Originality is the key to success although this has been hijacked a bit in recent times through manufactured boy and girl bands. When you think about the outstanding pop artists there are tell tale signs of their original minds. When not performing they often revert to their natural behaviour, which is one of living in seclusion away from other people. It might be thought that this is a reaction to the pressures of being in the limelight however this is how they should naturally behave in any case. The original family lived in seclusion away from other people in the original desert existence. Pop stars can demonstrate positive and negative obsessive behaviour in various forms be it the desire to feed starving people, buying large quantities of needless items or the taking of excessive amounts of illicit substances.

Other forms of creative entertainment include art and writing. The great artists are known for eccentric behaviour think of Van Gough, Picasso and De Vinci. Great writers

203

demonstrate the characteristics of the original mind. These people have learnt the art of story telling and without any natural constraints are able to take fiction beyond the limits of the tribal mind. Betrix Potter was eccentric and used to wear a sack over her head in the rain. She could easily have afforded an umbrella. Roald Dahl used to eat Norwegian prawns with mayonnaise and lettuce followed by a Kit Kat for lunch every day. He could have tried eggs for a change.

A further function that the shaman performed in his religious duties was that of teacher to the tribe. This gives us a further profession that exists today and that is the teaching profession. The character of the teacher again is naturally suited to the character of the original mind. Teachers spend their time telling rather than listening as part of the teaching process. They are there to tell the children how to do things like read and write. Teachers work alone with their class. Teachers can sometimes be a little on the eccentric side.

Following on from the shaman's religious work we have his everyday practical work. This work includes his being medic to the tribe. He provided for mental well being through religion but also provided for physical well being through his practical work as a doctor. Just think how many doctors have an abrasive bedside manner. This characteristic comes from evolution and reflects the lack of social skills from the original unsociable existence. Think how scruffy a doctor's handwriting can be. This comes from inferior coordination skills compared to those developed in the tribe through hunting with spears. Whilst these may not be desirable characteristics the original mind has characteristics that are essential for this area of work. A lack of compassion is essential in dealing with life and death decisions a doctor has to make. These decisions have to be made without human emotion clouding medical judgement. The doctor has to be able to cope with informing relatives of the death of loved ones. Only original minds have the natural ability to be able to cope with this and it is an essential ability in this area of work. Through an inferior natural level of coordination the surgeon develops a superior learnt level of coordination necessary for the intricate nature of surgery.

Next come the craftsmen. These were the sons of shamans. In the modern world craftsmanship has been somewhat superseded by the industrialists who were also original minds. The mass production of items by machine has meant that craftsmen are concentrated in specialised areas that mechanisation has yet to reach. One such area of work is the building trade. The craftsmen of the past were carpenters, stone masons and metal workers. They honed their skills over years of training and were specially regarded people. They provided their services first to the tribe and following on from this to the works created by the civilisations. It is civilisation that leads us to the next areas of work established by the original minds.

Civilisation required the establishment of artificial rules of behaviour and this lead to the creation of law. The legal system today is based on the thoughts of the original mind. The lack of prejudgement and logical questioning to try and arrive at truth are the basis of the system. If you think about it you will find there is no place in the legal system for tribal characteristics. Only symbols are used in the form of wigs and clothes to reflect the high status of the judge. This is a natural requirement of the tribal mind when it's being judged. The original mind should excel in this area of work if that is its area of interest. Barristers in a similar way to doctors are dealing with life altering decisions when they deal with criminal cases and the possibility of prison sentences. They again cannot be clouded with the emotion of compassion when defending or prosecuting cases. They have to be focussed on the law and evidence in cases to perform their function properly. If compassion got in the way criminals would be set free if they were nice people. I am not sure many are but there you are.

Along with the shaman's creation of personal wealth in the first classical civilisations came the establishment of the accountancy and banking. These professions are based on the original minds natural honesty. Honesty is a core necessity in declaring income to the tax man not that we clients always appreciate it. In banking, trust in the banker is essential in order for people to entrust their savings to him. Numerical ability is a characteristic of the original mind, which comes from the original farming existence when a natural ability at counting livestock meant survival.

Civilisation leads to demand for innovation and new ways of doing things. The craftsmen were the original innovators producing machines to make life easier. There was the invention of the wheel, boats, new types of building, new metals and all the other things that we recognise. Inventors today demonstrate the characteristics of the original mind. The typical perception of the inventor is one of eccentric behaviour with an obsessive personality. This character is essential in getting new ideas to work. The inventor needs to be unconcerned with people laughing at him and his new ideas. He needs obsession to see his ideas through to a conclusion. New things rarely work first time and it is only through correction and re-correction that something is made possible in the end.

Related to the inventor is the entrepreneur. This person makes new businesses work in a similar way to the inventor making inventions work. The entrepreneur also needs to demonstrate the character of the original mind. They demonstrate the ability to try new ways of doing things. They are not restricted like a tribal mind is by the natural thought that something can't be done. They demonstrate the obsession necessary to make new businesses work. They are risk takers but in a calculated way that should in theory lead to success. They don't always get it right but it's not a matter of life or death in the modern world.

As far as the tribal mind is concerned they fit into the businesses and structures created by original minds. There are certain positions that should naturally suit them. Staff Management is a particularly tribal reserve. Managers should naturally understand people and be able to organise them into a team. Mind you some of the ones I've met haven't been like this. The structure of management should appeal to the tribal mind. There is status in the various levels of management. The opportunity for career progression from junior to more senior positions creates motivation in the corporate structure just as it created motivation in the tribe. Management is all about personal relationships between managers themselves and between management and staff.

Another area of work that should suit the tribal mind is in sales. Selling is all about building personal relationships and understanding people and their desires. Today sales are generally geared towards the tribal mind, as it is this personality that forms the mass market. Evidence of this can be seen in the way products are sold. Cars for instance are produced in various levels of specification. The tribal mind aspires to the higher trim levels as an indication of their status in society. The Ghia trim level shows you are more successful than the LX trim level. It understands this and it takes the tribal mind to be able to communicate naturally with fellow minds. The sales man understands how the various complicated gadgets in cars will appeal to his status-orientated customer. He knows that his customer will show his new car to his next-door neighbour. The customer will need the best gadgets or he will face ridicule in the eyes of the neighbour. The salesman needs to be seen as a nice person. Honesty is not a characteristic that is essential in sales. A certain level of dishonesty is to be expected even if this is simply not pointing out faults with a car that is being sold. The salesman needs above all to be seen by the customer as someone like himself. This concept is tribal where being the same as other people in the tribe was essential for the group to function.

Chapter Twenty

Evolution of recreational behaviour

As primates sex is one of the most fundamental forms of recreational behaviour we have inherited and this comes from our evolution in the trees. That life gave us the instinct we would really like to indulge in but it is constrained by the instincts above it, practicality and the desire not to catch something nasty.

The order of lust

The most basic instinct is to have sex with as many partners as possible. This can be seen in some cultures where one man has lots women. Women do not seem to try and indulge this sort of activity although then perhaps I haven't met the right sort.

Following from this there is to have two women or men. This features in threesomes and foursomes. This behaviour evolved from the period in evolution of the clever running man.

The next instinct most deeply etched on our brains is to have just one partner because of affordability. Both man and women were needed to rear children because of the shortage of food.

The next instinct is both man and woman to have a few changeable partners and this came from the tribe. There was variety and the opportunity for greater choice than in the previous two periods of evolution. Greater sexual pleasure evolved along with sexual prowess.

In the last two instincts we see the split between the original and tribal minds.

In the tribe it would have been group sex and there's an interesting thought. It would be safer this way. If you nipped off for a bit you might have been eaten by a lion or something. This is unless of course you fancied the chief's bird and then it would be behind a bush unless you wanted to lose certain treasured assets. The size of the male appendage is likely to come from the tribe. Such equipment would be important as a way of showing women how much fun they could have. Any tribal bird that says she's not bothered is probably lying to make her bloke feel better. For the original mind in woman size shouldn't be much of an issue. The original man's missus didn't have much choice. She got what she was given. Could modern behaviour of the tribal mind not being able to resist other birds or blokes be a lot more natural than we would like to admit? Was monogamy the domain of the original mind and foisted on the tribal mind through religion?

For the original mind, I'm afraid things are somewhat duller in the sex department. I believe there could be a natural predisposition to premature ejaculation unfortunately. Sexual prowess came from the tribe. Circumcision seems to be used to try and match tribal superiority however the original mind shouldn't like bits being chopped off. The Karma Sutra could give a clue here. I think this may have been written by an original mind with a view to gaining competitive advantage. The original mind is adaptable and can find different ways around inadequacies. From inferiority is born superiority. The writing of the Karma Sutra would certainly have required somebody fairly obsessed with sex for all the ideas.

From my observations there is an obvious stumbling block for the teenage original boy in the pursuit of sex. That block is the simple fact that the tribal mind outnumbers the original mind by a good margin. If a tribal mind does stop long enough to take a look, and they may do, the original teenage mind will need a good theory in place. It needs to be born in mind that in the original existence there was no chatting up done because there was no language. The art of seduction by the whispering of sweet nothings into the ear of the girl was tribal. Therefore my view is that an original boy will need a theory. Now I have to say I am not an expert in this department other than I have come up with rather a lot of bad ones.

One of these theories was that fat birds up north should be less fussy. The logic is hopefully fairly obvious. I needed to try this theory out in the cultural capital for such things and so I went to Doncaster. It was a Saturday night and the club was full. I eyed the birds up for bulk. This was following several pints of lager it has to be said. Always better to try theories out with lager they do seem to compliment each other. Anyway the fattest bird wasn't interested and so I progressed my way down in bulk. I thought the theory was working as I arrived at the second fattest. She seemed quite interested. Not bad you might say. I tried my charms. It has to be said this theory is rubbish. Fat birds up north are just as fussy.

Another one of my theories was that birds should do what you want if they like you. There was unfortunately a crucial step I missed out in the application of this theory and that was the liking you bit. Getting pissed on a night out with the lads and throwing up on a bird the next day doesn't seem to work or ingratiate you to that bird's affections for some reason. I can't imagine why.

A theory that did seem to work was being obnoxious to the bird's parents. It was important to put ones feet on the coffee table and be thoroughly disliked. It was also essential to grunt rather than talk in a suitably teenage manner even though I was perhaps a bit old for it. The logic here was to create a rebel image. What is actually created is a rude obnoxious git image. I suspect it was more the wife's gullibility than the theory that worked here.

I will provide a few observations for the teenage girl with an original mind. Again they are heavily outnumbered. They won't naturally understand bitchiness, which is the tribal way of establishing order amongst girls. Dress sense may prove a tricky thing to get right. Remember if this story's right there should be no natural sense of dress code as there's no natural sense of self-image. Tribal girls establish this through selecting dress from the stars that they look up to. In the original existence there was nobody to look to and copy apart from the parents. In today's modern fashion world copying your mum's style might be a bit dodgy. The girl with an original mind will have to try and copy the tribal girl as best she can. She should try and remember not to forget her knickers. These could prove to be a deal breaker if she's after a tribal man. G-strings are in order, big pants are out. I know big pants are much more comfy. If she's after a boy with an original mind then it doesn't really matter. He won't be that fussy.

If an original girl becomes obsessed with her appearance as can happen when trying to fit in with the tribal ways this will need attention. It can get out of hand. She should naturally be looking for the connection that happens between original minds. Only they understand each other. Well some of the time any way. She is likely to be looking for a special level of commitment. The original man and his wife had this commitment. They had an intuition for each other and their relationship was for life for better or for worse.

If things don't quite go right as can happen on occasion the obsessive tendencies can manifest themselves in different ways. I have observed serial sexual encounters in an attempt to copy tribal ways. The tribal mind however doesn't usually have quite as many encounters as this. The original mind obsessed with sexual satisfaction may find itself on a road to nowhere or perhaps to some utopian bliss. Sexual pleasure increased in the tribe and the tribal mind. There was however a natural limit to the importance of sexual satisfaction. Whether the original mind can extend these limits into the unnatural and achieve greater satisfaction I am afraid I cannot say. It is possible and there are some bizarre practices in existence that don't altogether seem natural to me.

The other most basic form of recreational behaviour from our time in the trees is eating. Today this recreation takes the form of sitting in front of the TV with bags of crisps and boxes of chocs. Our inherited laziness means we do tend to get rather fat in our pursuit of this basic pleasure. In the past we at least had to climb a tree to get to our goodies, which gave us some exercise. Now we get in our cars and waddle around the shops. The extent of our effort is limited to opening packets, throwing away rubbish and going to the loo.

In the tribe we see evolution of the next level of leisure. By working together as a team large game could be killed which provided sufficient food to feed the tribe for a few days. This allowed time for recreation in between hunts. Recreation passed the time and also served to bond people together. Pleasure was taken in competing with fellow tribal members for fun. These pastimes also served to hone hunting skills with each tribal member competing to be the quickest runner or the best spear thrower. Strength would be tested and compared through wrestling contests. The tribal women would watch these contests of strength, speed and skill. The stronger, faster and more skilled the man the more sexually attractive he was in the eyes of the women.

Other recreation in the tribe included the development of ritual towards sex. Dance evolved whereby men and women would display themselves to each other through ritual movement. The existence of choice served to raise sexual stimulation. This mind evolved to have a natural sense of rhythm where the body would move in time to the beat of the drum. Sense of rhythm proved to be sexually stimulating and was selected for naturally in the tribe. It is likely I suspect that a good sense of rhythm probably indicates a good sense of rhythm and increased pleasure in sex.

The recreation of dining out at good restaurants originates from the tribe. The concept of nice food is tribal and it is actually a reflection of status. The head of the tribe got the best bits. This was probably an eyeball or some other delicacy from the kill. When we think of restaurants today status is very much part of dining out. There are restaurants that are exclusive and the ones to be seen in. There are tables in restaurants that are better than others. There are exclusive wines and expensive dishes. This is all about status rather than food in reality. The appreciation of good food and wine is an indicator of ones position in society. Those that choose based on volume of chips and quantity of lager are clearly of the lower orders. Cordon bleu cuisine along with the hundred quid bottle of wine is for those of the higher orders.

Team sports ought to appeal to the tribal mind rather than the original mind one might suspect. However we need to look in a little more detail at the team sports that exist. Football or soccer originated in Britain and so we might suspect that this game was created by the original mind. When we consider the game in detail we find that rather than natural cooperation we are looking at an artificial form of cooperation. The game has set rules to play by and specific positions for people to play in. Even the very act of kicking a ball around has no natural practical purpose. Kicking things around in the tribe served no function for hunting or impressing women. The game probably originated from some macabre warrior practice of kicking victim's heads around. It still has to be said this didn't impress women at least not the sort you wanted anyway. Football's appeal however is universal to both mind types. The team activity appeals naturally to the tribal mind. The obsession necessary to become a top player can appeal to the original mind.

Individual games may appeal to original minds and perhaps one of the oddest ones created is golf. Hitting a small ball with a stick quite clearly has no natural origin or purpose. This game has the appeal of tranquillity and walking which both reflect life in the original existence in the desert. The golf course offers space to the original mind, which it needs, particularly if it lives an urban existence.

The pastime of reading fiction ought to appeal to the tribal mind perhaps more so than the original mind. Stories originated with language and came from the tribe. The original mind can lack the patience necessary for reading a lengthy novel. It tends to prefer more factually based works of literature.

Boozing and smoking are a recreation for both minds as they access more basic body functions. The tribal mind will find appeal in the socialising aspect of the pub or bar. The original mind will find appeal in the consumption of large volumes of booze and the consequential effect it has in anaesthetising the mind.

One interesting area of fascination I have observed in the original mind is an interest in guns. I have known a few original minds that have had this hobby. The reason for this I believe is that the original mind innately doesn't like fighting because it's dangerous. It therefore likes to dominate any potential fight with superior technology, which is what guns represent. The reality is guns are rather dangerous especially if both potential combatants have them. I think this could be a link back in time to when Britain fought Africans and the Americans fought Indians. Then it was all right because only our sides had the guns. Certain guns do have a beauty in their design. The Colt 45 peacemaker is such a weapon. However the preferred choice of gun for the original mind would have been the blunderbuss or shotgun because the original mind is naturally a bad shot. These are represented today in the form of machine guns the ultimate weapon for the man who can't shoot straight.

Another area of interest to the original mind is sailing. Clearly relatively recent migration to Britain has involved sailing to get here however the interest seems to be deeper than simply getting over the Channel. This suggests to me that sailing and the original mind have had a close relationship in evolution and an interest in it has been genetically passed down through the generations. The story of Noah's Ark perhaps gives us an idea of where this might have originated. Is it possible for instance that people lived on the land currently under the Mediterranean Sea at the height of a cold phase in our ice age? As the world entered a warmer phase sea levels rose and spilled over from the Atlantic Ocean into the Mediterranean basin. This caused an immense flood. One or two original minds perhaps with guidance from God anticipated the flood and built arks to save themselves and their livestock. They survived by sailing to dry land and passed an interest in sailing on to their descendents. The story of this event was passed down through the generations and distorted with the passage of time. It would eventually culminate in the biblical story of Noah's Ark.

Chapter Twenty One

Psychology

What does our evolution mean for psychology? The answer is everything. Understand it and we understand why we behave as we do. I have approached the relative mystery of our evolution by looking at our current behaviour as was originally suggested by Charles Darwin in 1859. Darwin used classical observational methods to establish the process of natural selection. I believe his vision was one of similar methods being used to reveal the mysteries of the specifics of human evolution. The scientific study of human behaviour has had nearly one hundred and fifty years since then to find *"the origin of man and his history"* with rather little to show for our efforts. Why is this? I suspect the reason lies in the nature of the study of psychology.

I managed to last two weeks of a degree course in psychology at Sheffield University. For me there was too much animal cruelty involved. The keeping of kittens in boxes and the electrocution of dogs offend the original mind's close connection with animals. It is the original innovative mind that is capable of making new discoveries and it has a sensitive nature particularly towards animal cruelty. More fundamentally much of the basis for our current understanding came from a time when eugenics was part of human philosophy. Today we can divorce such thinking from science however at the time that people were working on the initial observations of autism eugenics was part of the current thinking. There was a normal personality and variation from that was abnormal; however perhaps they were wrong. There wasn't in fact a single normal human personality but rather two.

The research that I studied in my two weeks centred on distinguishing between innate or inherited behaviour and learnt behaviour. Both of these behaviours have their origins in natural behaviour. Learnt behaviour came from somewhere going right back to man's first use of tools. The hand axe had its origin in a naturally occurring tool and that was the tooth. Human group behaviour had its origin in naturally occurring groups of people. Had we all lived in single families we would not have human social ability. Had we all lived in tribes we would not now have single families.

Psychiatry is about the treatment of mental disorders. It is in effect repairing broken psychology. To repair something it is always useful to know how it works and to know this we need to know the mind's evolution. In effect how it was made. Once we know this we are in a position to know what to repair. There is little point in trying to repair something that isn't broken.

Should I venture into the world of psychiatry? I know I shouldn't I have no medical qualifications. However I am proposing a new manual on the workings of the human mind and so I think a little dabbling is in order don't you? I will however endeavour to limit myself as best I can.

First we will take Asperger's Syndrome. Can this be cured? This is a patently ridiculous proposition to me. Its like saying can a black man be cured of being black. Of course not! There is nothing to cure. The original mind is different from the tribal mind as a matter of race in just the same way as modern Africans are a different race to white Europeans. The split in race of the mind occurred before the split in skin colours however it is no less a matter of race. Thinking differently is no different to looking different just harder to spot perhaps or not in some cases.

Should behaviour be modified? In my view only in so far as is necessary. Everybody's natural behaviour has to be modified to some extent to fit in with modern society. Our society is a creation born out of concepts from both mind types. We have social behaviour from the tribal mind and individual behaviour from the original mind. Neither is completely suited to the modern world and each has to compromise to some extent. This compromise in my view should be in the interests of personal happiness and for the avoidance of going to prison.

One of the most significant human characteristics that can cause problems is obsession. Obsession was born out of need in evolution. Those that developed obsession survived. In the tribe obsession was watered down by natural selection in order that a tribe of people could function together. For the original mind this was not the case as there was no social behaviour that needed it to be so. It is therefore the original mind that is likely to suffer from obsession related problems.

Obsessive behaviour may have served a purpose in evolution however now it can be obsolete in certain circumstances. It is useful and essential to write long waffling theories however if you are not engaged in such things it may find itself surfacing where it is not wanted. Obsessive compulsive behaviour takes all sorts of forms be it with personal hygiene, lying, anorexia, tidiness, phobias, collecting too many things and the list goes on. Underneath is obsession. Obsession as a characteristic cannot be cured because of its natural programming in the original mind. It may however be diverted into more positive uses and the psychiatrist is there to help with the diversion.

Autism in the classical sense is debilitating and something that causes us great fear. I believe it is the original mind that is vulnerable to autism and it is triggered by stress induced external influences. This could be through trauma, illness or by inoculation. It would seem that the mind is accelerated beyond a point of no return and remains in that accelerated state. Functions that facilitate learning in normal minds are shut down as the mind looks to within itself and the influence of external sources is limited. This can give a greater inward mental ability; however there are often no ways of properly expressing those thoughts.

Communication abilities fail to be learnt and can even be lost. In the event of original mental characteristics being demonstrated by the parents I would be careful of risks that may trigger originally minded children being tripped over into an autistic state. I have personally managed to take my own mind close to what seemed similar to autism on one occasion and it was not at all nice. The mind will just not stop no matter what you seem to do.

Schizophrenia is very similar in many ways to Asperger's Syndrome and is really only a slight variation from the original personality. The symptoms of schizophrenia that vary from the basic normal characteristics are delusions and hallucinations. It is a natural characteristic of the original personality to be able to convince itself that something is real. This can be an imaginary friend or voices from God or some other things that might seem a bit odd. The common view of schizophrenia is that of the split personality as illustrated in the story "Dr Jekel and Mr Hide". In effect we all do have two personalities. One is natural and one is leant. If we alter from one to the other in a substantial way a split personality can be seen. We may be sociable through learnt behaviour yet at another time revert to our natural anti sociable habits.

One of my favourite mental disorders is that of Narcissistic Personality Disorder. In brief the Narcissist is somebody who is obsessed with their own importance. They can think they are fantastic in bed, super clever, extremely powerful, extremely attractive and various other self-important visions. I suspect a narcissistic client naffed off a narcissistic psychiatrist and led to this classification. The disorder describes the original mind and arises if that mind unfortunately isn't quite as good as he thinks he is. If he is as good as he thinks he is then he is the boss and it's all right to be like this. Many of the outstanding people in history had characteristics of narcissism. Nelson adorned his home with pictures of himself. Napoleon thought he was an emperor and could conquer Europe. The expectation of human modesty and natural self-image

219

comes from the tribal mind. For the original mind there are no such natural constraints. As such people with original minds substitute an artificial modesty and self-image of themselves in place of a natural view. Combine this with obsession we have somebody who can think he is better than he is. It may be that this person perhaps is as good as he thinks - its just nobody else does and then we have the narcissist.

In Japan there is phenomenon called Taijin Kyofusho. I call it a phenomenon but it isn't really it is simply an observation of the original mind functioning in a social environment or not as the case may be. Taijin Kyofusho is a fear of basically causing offence to others. This fear is born out of a natural lack of self-awareness in the original mind. Artificial behaviour steps into this void and as has been seen this leads to a wide variety if that behaviour is purely learnt especially when combined with obsession. Japan is culturally a polite society. In a similar way to polite society in Britain in the eighteenth and nineteenth centuries, cultural behaviour can become a little extreme. Britain during that period took politeness to a point that we find entertaining today. In Japan Taijin Kyofusho is an over reaction to a culture which has become unnaturally polite. Japan does have a character that would indicate a concentration of original minds. It is an island just as Britain is an island. This makes it a refuge for the displaced rather than a prime central area that tribes would compete to hold. The Japanese are an innovative people and as with other original minds problems with obsession can surface.

Attention Deficit Disorder seems to be more common now in children that it used to be. This is a process of the original mind running too quickly for decisions to be remembered. What I think happens here is that a decision is taken but before it can be properly stored in the memory the mind has already moved onto the next decision. The cure is to slow the mind down and presumably this is what drugging it does. I have to say I am not a big fan of using drugs because the original mind has a bit of taste for them and starting it early in my view is perhaps not the best thing to do.

The cause of attention deficit disorder is in my view from living a lifestyle that is unnaturally interesting. When I was a lad things were a lot less stimulating than they are now. We would have the test card to watch on the television. Where has that gone I ask? It was most therapeutic and uninteresting. Food was all home prepared without any interesting additives to get you going. Computer games had just been invented and involved a dot being knocked from one side of the TV to the other. It needs to be considered that in the original desert existence pretty much nothing interesting happened at all. There was the excitement of catching the odd not very tasty lizard and that was about it. Prior to this there was the time of the clever running man and that was more interesting however not really for the children as they lived in the mountains away from the excitement. Today we have excitement and stimulation all the time and it isn't natural. We are addicted to excitement and it isn't good for us.

I do see a difficulty in drawing the line between what might be considered autistic in the classical sense and normal in the Asperger sense. The characteristics are the same it is the ability to take on learnt behaviour that is the difference. We can only really tell this after the opportunity to learn has happened. Current thought is with a view to early classification with a view to early intervention. The problem with this approach is you can't really tell except with the obvious cases. The obvious is where no language is being learnt. For everybody else the rate of learning will vary. For some people it may take their whole lives to pick up tribal characteristics. Others may pick them up quicker. It is my view that intervention should be restricted to the obvious. One thing we shouldn't do is remove the opportunity to learn. At the moment I perceive that this is exactly what is happening in the rather liberal use by schools of one to ones on children perceived as having

Asperger's Syndrome. If exposure to tribal behaviour is missed in the formative years of a child it may well never recover those years of learning with greater problems simply being stored up for the future. In adulthood we can't go round with a one to one protecting us. Much greater effort needs to be devoted to forming bonds of friendship for these children to provide them with the protection they need in school. Further answers lie in pressing society back towards the original natural values of honesty, clarity, simplicity and order.

Chapter Twenty Two

Philosophy

Until recently life has been relatively mundane and ordered for most of the time. We had a society based on class structure. It wasn't common to move between classes and as such people for better or worse knew where they were and what to expect. There was predictability and almost inevitability to one's fate. We had religion to guide our behaviour. What have we got now? Endless possibilities and choices! We have no set social structure any more and religion has virtually no influence on most people's lives.

If it is properly understood why we behave as we do we can develop a belief and use it to find the way forward. Belief is something that is lacking in Western Society at the moment especially here in Britain. We are looking for it and I believe we need to fully understand ourselves to find it. That belief needs to be what we should do to make us more content. No longer is belief in science or technology enough for us. These things don't provide the answers. They are the modern day equivalent of false Gods. We need a new belief based on understanding our own minds.

This belief needs to reflect both types of mind, as one needs the other. We need innovation from the original mind and social values from the tribal mind. Each has to restrain the other from going too far. At the moment in Britain the original mind needs to reassert itself. The tribal mind is consuming too much in the desperate attempt to achieve status. There is so much stuff now how can status be achieved? Everybody's got that stuff anyway.

My view is that we need to try and mirror the original way of life as closely as we can. That means different things for different people. For the tribal mind that means trying to mirror the tribal existence. Work and home life need to be on a tribal scale with the personal interactions the tribe would have had. The original mind needs to find itself space, tranquillity and control over its life.

There needs to be simplification of most things that exist today for the benefit of everybody. We were not programmed in evolution for the current level of complexity that we have to deal with. Tax is super complicated with Family Tax Credit, Working Tax Credit, Child Tax Credit, Income Tax along with a multitude of other taxes and credits. We have multiple utility providers. We have more laws than we know what to do with. We have multiple remote controls for the TV, video and DVD that seem to compete with each other not to be found. Cars have thief proof wheels, which unfortunately seem to also be change proof when you get a flat tyre. I could go on but then I am starting to sound like my Gran complaining about inflation in the nineteen seventies.

The philosophy is simple - look back at our evolution understand it and thereby understand ourselves.

Chapter Twenty Three

Summary

I will summarise the evolutionary journey that I have set out and just take a look at the alternative path that may have been available at what I consider to be the critical later point in human evolution.

In the beginning the human ancestor evolved from the sea to become a small insectivore creature driven fear. These fears are real and relived by children in their bedrooms at night. We first ran from giant spiders and evolved to hide later from dinosaurs. These monsters are set out in mythology from all corners of the earth. The dragon was a pterosaur or flying reptile. The human ancestor was prey to this monster and survived through developing fear of this creature. Home was the rock crevice, which was a place of safety until the creature we most associate with evil evolved to hunt us in our home. This creature is the snake and he was a monster that would find us and kill us in our beds. The snake caused us to fear the dark and tights spaces, which would in turn lead us to a new life in the canopy of the forest.

In the canopy of the forest we evolved our primate form. We turned from a nocturnal existence into a creature that was active in the day. We needed to see to climb in the trees. Colour vision evolved to identify the fruit that now became our staple diet. It would be on this diet that we would grow into much larger creatures. We would become lazy, self-indulgent pleasure seeking animals and our greed would be our downfall from this utopian existence. We still resent our greed now for this downfall and it came about through our growing too large to climb safely in the canopy of the forest. We developed the fear of heights through seeing fellow ancestors fall and die, which would make us into ground living hominoids.

It is now that we consider divergent paths for our evolution. We know that from finds of hominoid remains so far that we were the last to emerge from the central area of origin in East Africa. This means that according to my principle that *"the most competitive creature holds the original central territory"* we were the most competitive hominoid. This is further supported by the fact we are the only species of hominoid alive today. The alternative to the path of evolution that I have set out is the conventional view that we evolved as a cooperative species and that it was social cooperation that made us the most competitive of species. On a simple basis this is a tempting view to take. There are however too many anomalies in current human behaviour to fit in with this view.

Had we all evolved from a cooperative tribe we would not have the natural single-family unit of a man a woman and children. We would all live as nature intended in a tribal group. Most of us don't live in this way. If everybody were naturally cooperative we would not have what is termed Asperger's Syndrome. Had the tribal group been the only natural form of group structure we would not have the concept of Adam and Eve and monogamy. Had there only been the tribe we would not have personal wealth and capitalism. For me the conventional view of us all evolving from a tribal group just does not fit how we behave today. The single family of a man woman and children is the foundation stone of human group behaviour. This sized group was formed by evolution.

With the single-family group structure forming the foundation of human behaviour we have anti social behaviour propelling us towards this sized group. We see a break down in cooperation between the hominoid ancestors of men. The split in the hominoid tree that would lead to Homo sapiens was born out of a human characteristic that we have inherited and that is the ability to run. Running is conventionally thought to have arisen out of competition with animals. This view however does not fit for the simple reason that four legs are always

226

faster than two legs unless they are attached to a tortoise. The animals of the African plains are all faster than a man could ever be. Running ability evolved from competition with relative hominoid species. Rather than running after relative hominoids we evolved to run away from them. This behaviour is demonstrated through childhood games. The games are hide and seek and tag along with an accompanying fear of the bogie man. We became prey to relative hominoids and so evolved to become isolated clever running men.

The process of natural selection chose the best individuals for survival. It was through this process that Homo sapiens evolved to be individually superior to relative hominoids. They were cooperatively superior; however when we came to the time of great austerity in East Africa they could not survive in their larger group structures in the desert. This environment could only support single-family units who were widely spread out. Homo sapiens held on in this environment through obsessively searching for food. The best were naturally selected and perhaps at this time God did look down on us and make the decision that we as a species should survive with his guidance.

As the environment returned from desert to savannah so evolved the tribe of men. With it evolved the tribal mind and tribal behaviour. The original family however did not die out but rather evolved to become a farmer. This would create an instinct to farm and a close mental connection with animals. The wide spread nature of farming that emerged around 10,000 years BC suggests that farming developed as an instinct much earlier than convention thinks, prior to the migration out of Africa. So we come to cooperation between the original family and the tribe. This arose out of need and gave us the concept of the offering by the tribe to the original family. This offering would form a foundation for religious worship and a reverence for the original family. Original minds would become part of the tribe and form special positions for themselves. This started with the shaman as religious leader, which became a privileged position within the tribe.

As the tribes migrated from Africa with original people in their number there emerged an excess of original minds. Because of a lack of natural cooperative ability and a limit on the number of special positions within the tribe these people became the unwanted and the displaced. Some would find a life in the north as warriors in the Neanderthal Wars and their descendents would form the warrior cultures. The tribes fought; however the warrior evolved out of a war of annihilation. It was from this that the concept of war came to be. Other original minds were pressed out through competition with the tribes to the places where the first classical civilisations would emerge. Civilisation evolved through people congregating together who did not naturally have cooperative skills. In place of natural rules of cooperative behaviour would evolve artificial rules of behaviour and so is created civilisation.

The geographic human structure of the world would be formed through further migration with original minds flowing out of the original central areas to the peripheries. One of these migrations was through Britain and on to America and Australia. These final countries of migratory destination have the greatest concentrations of original minds with the original central area of the in East Africa having the greatest concentration of tribal minds.

And so there we have the story of human evolution and the cause of the autistic personality. Understand them and we have an understanding of the human world of today.

Chapter Twenty Four

Conclusion

I believe that we each need to understand our own minds and this process should be one of self-reflection. We have a spectrum of predictable human personalities. At one end we have original minds and the other end tribal minds. In the middle we have I believe the hybrid mind, which is a mixture of the two. This mind is perhaps the most difficult one to decipher with elements of each basic form of behaviour working together or possibly conflicting with each other.

We certainly all have conflicting natural behavioural programming from earlier evolution. At one time we were very promiscuous and at another monogamous. At one time we were active at night and at another in the day. At one time we ate fruit and at another meat. At one time we had a lot to eat and another very little to eat. Once we were the hunted and at another time we were the hunter. At one time we were lazy self-indulgent creatures and at another obsessive workers. Confused - well I think that is perfectly natural considering our evolution.

Is there a perfect existence that we can aspire too? I am afraid there is not! 3 or 4 billion years of evolution cannot be undone. Conflict will always exist within the human mind. One layer of evolutionary programming will conflict with another layer. This conflict makes complete satisfaction impossible to achieve. You could try having sex with a hundred different women but then you feel guilty about cheating on the wife. If you didn't feel guilty I'm sure the wife would ensure that you did by one means or the other. You can stay monogamous and not feel guilty but think of all those lovely women you are missing. You can try being lazy but then you will feel guilty for not doing anything. You can try working hard but all the time you would rather loaf around. There is no answer to how you achieve perfect satisfaction and therein lays the answer - you can't. There are however ways to get closer to it if never actually achieving it and so we will set that out instead.

With a knowledge of your own mind you should have a better idea of what you should do to make yourself more content. Trying to do something your mind isn't suited to may be doomed to failure. For the original mind this means networking and parties may always be unpleasant and perhaps best avoided. There's no disgrace in this - who wants to be nice and boring. For the tribal mind trying to copy the innovative thought patterns of the original mind is likely to be doomed to failure. There is no disgrace in this. Innovation isn't all it's cracked up to be. It's actually rather unpleasant and self-destructive.

For children with original minds I think they may need to know why they are like they are. They don't have a dysfunction and do not need persecuting by tribal or other original minds because they are different and sometimes a bit tricky to handle. By telling these children they have something wrong with them they will believe they have something wrong with them and they don't. They do need to be part of society because it's their ancestors that formed society. They may need a little guidance in recognising tribal characteristics however I feel they shouldn't be set so far apart that they haven't the opportunity to naturally learn these values from their fellow children. This learning is essential for their future life. These children will be the future leaders and think where we would be if all the past great people had been told they had something wrong with them. If Winston Churchill had been excluded from school for destroying the Head Master's hat we may all be goose-stepping now.

For the world of work it may be helpful to understand yourself. By understanding your mind you will have a better understanding of the sort of work that will suit you. You will further have a better understanding of the kind of position that will suit you better. Should you wish to occupy a position that you are naturally not suited for you will need to learn the abilities necessary for that position. As far as the original mind is concerned it is capable of learning all the tribal characteristics provided that is what it wants to do. It does need to remember however that these characteristics shouldn't be taken too far. As for the tribal mind being able to unlearn natural tribal behaviour I am not sure that this altogether possible or desirable. It will however have to take on original values if it wishes to work in the professions created by the original mind.

For the world it would help if countries understood why other countries have different values to theirs. The balance of mind types is different from one country to the next. This balance dictates a country's culture and those countries where original minds have concentrated will naturally have different values to those where tribal minds are concentrated. Tribal culture should tend towards better social awareness provided its not ruled by some despot dictator. Unfortunately tribal countries are more prone to dictatorship due to a lack of numbers of original minds to oppose the one in power. Western cultures and particularly that of the USA are geared towards original values. These values are capitalist and centre on individual family well being, rather than the well being of the community. I can see no reason for the West to try and impart its values on anybody else. It's much better to keep these things to ourselves. Wealth doesn't create contentment of the mind and also tends to burn up rather a lot of oil. There's only so much to go around.

The fundamental question that has to be asked is this story right? Are our fears from where I say they are from? The conventional thought about human evolution that I have read always seems to envisage us in a similar physical form to that we have today. Furthermore conventional thought always seems to envisage us as sociable and we evolved as sociable creatures.

What I am suggesting may be different to that thought but then that is how the original innovative mind works. Can you imagine your ancestor in a completely different form to yourself? Can you imagine your ancestor as a tiny mouse like creature pressing himself into the depths of the rock crevice looking out at a dragon? Can you imagine life as a single family desperately searching for food in an arid desert? Can you imagine that rather than there being a single human mind there are actually two basic types of human mind? Can you imagine that it is in fact the existence of two minds that explains the world we live in today? This requires quite a lot of imagination I know. Could the story be proved or disproved?

What needs to be born in mind is this. Be it a scientist, theorist, artist or religious prophet we are trying to do the same thing. We are all trying to paint a picture that people will recognise. The scientist has a special level of credibility in Western society because of our cultural evolution through the industrial revolution. I believe that we have placed too much burden on the scientist to find the answers. We need to step back and look at the whole picture of humanity. Is the picture that I have painted one that you can recognise? I accept it could be better, have more detail and may have bits that are wrong. Things can always be better but then you never finish. Can you see the picture that I have painted?

For me the story makes logical sense. We as human beings rely on logic and things making sense. My conclusion is that there are two types of basic human mind that make up the human race. There is the tribal mind or conventional mind and there is the original mind or the mind observed by Hans Asperger. Both are normal and arise from different periods of evolution. Each has survived to the modern day and gives us the reason for the human world we live in today.

And so to the final question! Did God create man through evolution? Did he role the dice of life to see what would come up? Did he like what he saw in mankind and save us from extinction? Those are questions for you to answer for yourself.

232

Bibliography and Reference Material

For the most part this book is written from what I feel is common sense. I appreciate that my interpretation of the term may only be common to me at the moment; however I think you will find what I have said does make sense and so eventually it may become "common sense". There are a few literatures that have helped me in arriving at my conclusions and they are set out below. I acknowledge with gratitude those authors and works.

Bibliography

Brown (Rev John): The Self-Interpreting Bible containing the Old and New Testaments: Date unknown.

Darwin (Charles): The Origin of Species: 1859.

Day, (M.H.): The Fossil History of Man. Oxford University Press. Burlington, NC. 1977.

Donald (J) and Blake (E): From Lucy to Language. Simon and Schuster 1996.

Frith (Uta): Autism and Asperger Syndrome: Cambridge University Press 1991.

Knopp (Guido): Hitler's Children: Sutton Publishing 2000.

Lifton (Robert Jay): The Nazi Doctors. Medical killing and the Psychology of Genocide. ISBN 0-465-09094. 1986.

Punshon (John): Portrait in Grey. a short history of the Quakers: Quaker Home Service. London 1984.

Roberts (J.M): The Earliest Men and Women: Book Club Associates. 1980.

References

Adams (Jonathan): Africa During the Last 150,000 Years: Environmental Sciences Division, Oak Ridge National Laboratory, USA. 2005.

American Psychiatric Association: Is Taijin Kyofusho a Culture Bound Syndrome? The American Journal of Psychiatry 160:1358, July 2003.

Asperger (H): Die "Autistischen Psychopathen" im Kinder: Archiv fur Psychiatrie und Nervenkrankheiten Pg 76-136. 1944.

Barondess (Jeremiah A): MD Care of the Medical Ethos: Reflections on Social Darwinism, Racial Hygiene and the Holocaust. 1/12/1988 Annals of Internal Medicine Vol 129 issue 11 part 1 pages 891-898.

Humphrey (N): Cave art, autism and the evolution of the human mind: Centre for Philosophy of Natural and Social Science at the London School of Economics 1998

Huxley (T) Life and Letters of Thomas Henry Huxley, Vol 1. London: p.170 Macmillan 1900

Journal of the American Medical Association (JAMA) 112 (1939) page 1981"The New Wiener Medizinische Gesellschaft" and "THE NAZI CREED WITH REGARD TO MEDICINE"

JAMA 109, 1937 page 1465

JAMA 101, 1933 page 866

JAMA 113, 1939 page 1501

Roach (John): Fear of Snakes, Spiders Rooted in Evolution : National Geographic News 04/10/2001.

White, T, G.Suwa, and B. Asfaw. 1994. Australopithecus ramidus, a new species of early hominoid from Aramis, Ethiopia. Nature volume. 371.pp. 306-312 also volume. 375 pg. 88.

Printed in the United Kingdom
by Lightning Source UK Ltd.
119895UK00003B/235-243